The Easy Anti-Inflammatory Diet Cookbook

100 Fast and Simple Anti-Inflammatory Diet Recipes to Heal the Immune System and Live Longer

STEPHANIE TRASK

Copyright © 2018 Stephanie Trask

All rights reserved. No part of this publication may be reproduced, distributed, or transmitted in any form or by any means, including photocopying, recording, or other electronic or mechanical methods, without the prior written permission of the publisher, except in the case of brief quotations embodied in critical reviews and certain other noncommercial uses permitted by copyright law.

Limit of Liability/Disclaimer of Warranty: While the publisher and author have used their best efforts in preparing this book, they make no representations or warranties with respect to the accuracy or completeness of the contents of this book and specifically disclaim any implied warranties of merchantability or fitness for a particular purpose. No warranty may be created or extended by sales representatives or written sales materials. The advice and strategies contained herein may not be suitable for your situation. You should consult with a professional where appropriate. Neither the publisher nor author shall be liable for any loss of profit or any other commercial damages, including but not limited to special, incidental, consequential, or other damages.

ISBN-13: 978-1721090860

ISBN-10: 172109086X

DEDICATION

To all who desire to live life to the fullest!

TABLE OF CONTENT

INTRODUCTION

The immune system is one of the most complex and incredible elements of the human body and it is able to identify alien presence, which includes bacteria and viruses that may be harmful to the body. The immune system is sub-divided into two major parts, such as the innate immune system and the adaptive immune system. You were born with a completely intact innate immunity at birth, which comes with a defensive barricade like stomach acid and mucus. The innate immune system keeps out every outside threat such as cough reflex, fevers and many other antigens.

As you keep growing and developing in life, the adaptive immune system grows, adapts and develops also. Each exposure to an illness or germ is carefully documented by the adaptive immune system and this helps the body put together an automatic defense against such an illness or germ whenever you get exposed to it. An intricate system of cells, chemicals and biological pathways are used to achieve this adaptive immune process.

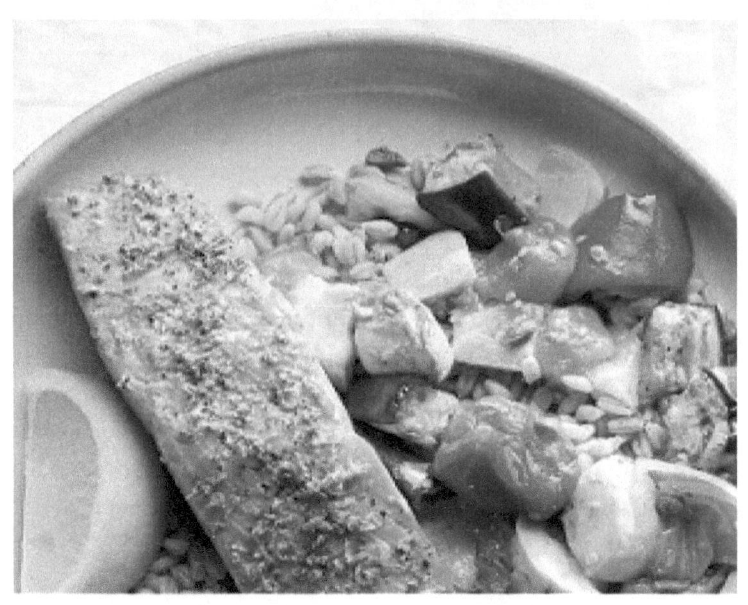

Inflammation and the Immune System

The inflammatory process is a very normal function of the body. The immune system activates inflammation to control tissue damage or an intruder when a potential threat is recognized. Chemical mediators known as cytokines act as indicator for the enlistment of other immune system parts which speed up the healing process by bringing about inflammation. Different proteins and cells such as white blood cells are stimulated by the immune system to restore damaged tissues and get rid of intruders and potential threats.

The inflammatory process is an integral part of the general healing process, including the healing of wounds and it is also a helpful system for getting rid of intruding microorganisms. Inflammation and the immune system go hand in hand, allowing helpful antibodies to enter into the needed area and stimulate other crucial parts of the immune system's response to speed up the healing process.

The inflammatory process of response is a succession of defense signals and systems that take on anti-inflammatory cells to the damaged area, which sequentially activates other cells that trigger other defensive systems and the like. The swelling and pain associated with inflammation are only an over-magnified response to threat or harm.

Immune System Dysfunction and Autoimmune Disease

The immune system can cause extreme or unnecessary inflammation if it gets compromised or out of control. The immune system has the ability to read distress signals (a protein known as antigen) on the surface of various cells, interpret the signal and effectively launch an attack if the cell is a likely harmful virus or bacteria. When the immune system loses part of its ability to differentiate between healthy and unhealthy cells; it is said to be dysfunctional. When the immune system becomes overactive or defective, it begins to attack healthy cells and tissues which culminate to autoimmune disease. Inflammation is a form of protection in a healthy immune system, but when it becomes defective or overactive, the inflammatory turns on healthy cells and tissues in the body instead of invaders.

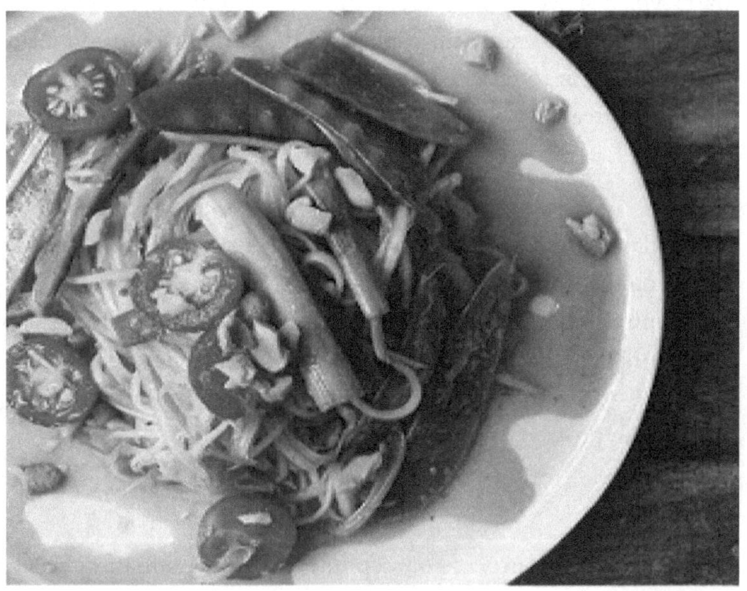

Inflammatory Types

Inflammation can be helpful or harmful to the body; consequently, it becomes important to understand the difference between acute and chronic inflammation. Acute inflammation happens inside a few minutes to hours with noticeable symptoms such as pain and swelling. Usually, the pain, swelling and redness that are experienced are a controlled reaction that will leave as healing takes place. This kind of inflammatory response is a sign of healing and healthy restoration of the body.

Alternatively, chronic inflammation is an indication of a more severe underlying condition with much less obvious signs. This inflammation type tends to linger for several days, weeks, and for years if not treated and it is very likely to lead to continuous and severe tissue damage and inflammatory diseases. Chronic inflammation has been connected to rheumatoid arthritis, obesity, heart disease, asthma and other severe medical conditions.

Chronic Inflammatory Symptoms

Although, chronic inflammatory signs can be subtle, there are revealing indications to know if you have chronic inflammation, including:

Mood swings

Gum disease

Excess weight and obesity

Fatigue and constant weakness

Rashes

Joint pain

Digestive problems such as bloating

Brain fog and recurrent headaches

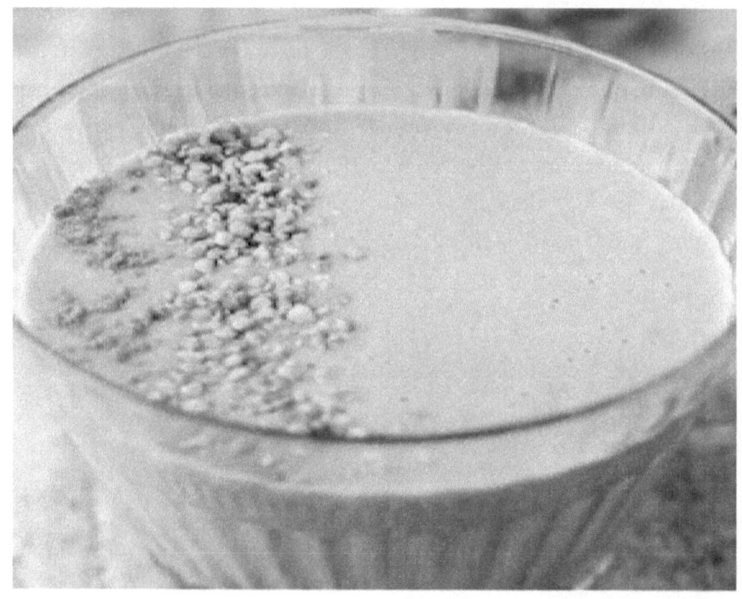

Diet and Chronic Inflammation

Certain food types have been known to cause inflammation and some other foods are known to fight and reduce inflammation. Diet is an important key in the fight against chronic inflammation. If you are suffering from an inflammatory or autoimmune condition, here are some common foods that cause inflammation:

Alcohol

Alcohol is a major cause of several disorders, medical conditions and diseases; and many of these diseases and medical conditions are related to inflammation.

Artificial Ingredients

MSG and aspartame are artificial ingredients that can trigger chronic inflammation.

Casein and Dairy

Lactose allergy or sensitive can be a contributing factor to inflammation. Dairy also contains casein proteins which have a comparable structure to gluten, which can be a threat to gluten-sensitive people and cause inflammation.

Gluten

The immune system of people with celiac disease or that are sensitive to gluten will take gluten protein as a potential threat; an immune response will be launched that will attack the intestines, causing nutrients malabsorption, and if left unchecked can lead to autoimmune disorders.

Refined Carbs

Refined carbs such as cookies, pasta, cakes etc, can contribute to inflammation.

Trans Fats and Saturated Fats

Systemic inflammation can be caused by consuming trans-fats. Tissue inflammation can be caused by the consumption of saturated fats which contributes to sever chronic inflammation and heart disease.

Sugar

Inflammatory pathways in the body can be induced by inflammatory chemical prompts caused by sugar consumption.

Your way of life is equally as important as your dietary choices. Attaining excellent health calls for a suitable anti-inflammatory diet, avoiding unwarranted stress, habitual exercise {30-60minutes, 4 or more times weekly} and getting enough sleep. The anti-inflammatory diet with some basic daily-life changes will help you prevent the risk of severe health problems caused by inflammation. You can enjoy a stress-free and better life with little or no illnesses.

Anti-Inflammatory Diet Tips

Chronic inflammation directly or indirectly contributes to many diseases and severe medical conditions, such as: cancer, Parkinson's disease, Alzheimer's disease, heart disease, rheumatoid arthritis and osteoarthritis. The drastic reduction and elimination of inflammation is possible and one major way it can be achieved is through dietary choices. Eating a diet that is anti-inflammatory will help to fight chronic inflammation, protect the body against a number of diseases, increase metabolism, stabilize blood sugar and sequentially slow the process of aging. Here are few anti-inflammatory diet tips to consider for optimal health:

- Eat a fiber rich diet that is rich in phytonutrients found in whole foods, whole grains (like oatmeal and barley) veggies (such as onions, eggplants and okra) and fruits (such as blueberries and bananas). Eat not less than 25g of fiber daily.

- Consume 4 servings of crucifers and alliums per week. Crucifers such as Brussels sprouts, mustard greens, cauliflower, cabbage and broccoli; and alliums, including leek, onions, scallions and garlic. Consuming at least 4 servings of crucifers and alliums can help lower cancer susceptibility.

- Eat surplus amounts of veggies and fruits. Eat not less than 9 servings of veggies and fruits daily. 1 serving equals 1 cup of a raw leafy veggie or 1/2 cup cooked veggie or fruit. For extra antioxidant properties, add spices and herbs, such as ginger and turmeric to your cooked veggies and fruits.

- Eat foods that are rich in Omega-3 fatty acids, such as soy beans, kidney beans, navy beans, walnuts and flax meal. You can also eat cold water fish such as anchovies, sardines, trout, mackerel, herring, oysters and salmon. You can also take high quality omega-3 supplements.

- Consume less saturated fat. Saturated fat should be reduced to not more than 10% of your total calories per day. Reduced saturated fat will limit heart disease risk. Red meat should also be limited to once weekly, and should be well marinated with unsweetened fruit juices, tart, spices and herbs to limit toxic compound that forms while cooking.

- Use healthy oils while cooking, such as organic expeller-pressed canola oil, extra virgin olive oil, expeller pressed high-oleic versions of safflower oil and sunflower oil.

- Consume low fat fish such as cold water fish and low fat fish such as flounder and sole that are filled with healthy fats.

- Avoid refined sugars and sweeteners, processed foods and foods high in sodium or containing high-fructose corn syrup. These foods contribute to chronic inflammation.

- Consume healthy snacks such as, walnuts, almonds, pistachios, carrots, celery sticks, unsweetened or plain Greek-style yogurt and fruits.

- Add spices (like thyme, sage, ginger, rosemary, turmeric, cinnamon and cloves) to your food and sweetened with phytonutrients filled fruits, such as carrots, berries, apricots and apples.

- Eliminate trans-fat from your diet, research show that trans-fat contributes to inflammation. Avoid foods that contain partially hydrogenated or hydrogenated oils, such as cookies, crackers, some margarines and veggie shortenings.

The anti-inflammatory diet is a guideline to help you achieve good health, a healthy immune system, overall wellbeing and longevity. With this new found knowledge and the recipes below, you can satisfactorily combat chronic inflammation, inflammatory conditions and autoimmune disorders.

Anti-Inflammatory Recipes

Breakfast

Flaxseed Banana and Zucchini Muffins

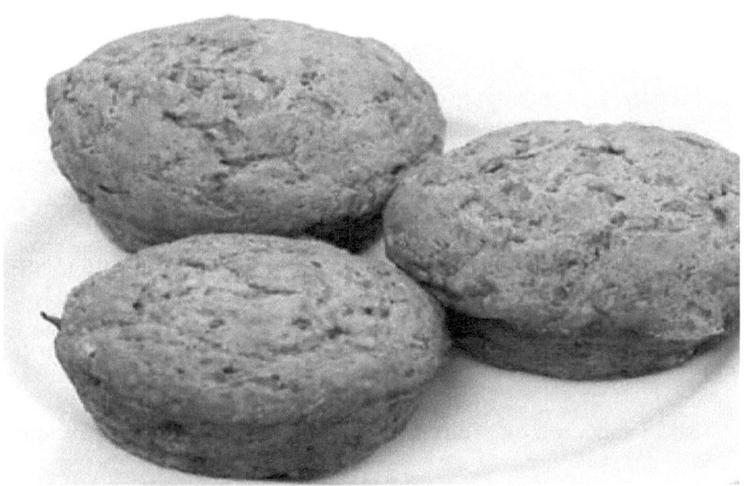

Preparation Time: 10 minutes

Cook Time: 25 minutes

Serves: 12 muffin servings

Ingredients

1 tsp baking powder

2 tsps baking soda

1 tsp cinnamon, ground

1/2 tsp sea salt

1 ripe big banana, mashed

1 1/2 cups zucchini, roughly grated

1 (lightly beaten) big egg

3/4 cup whole milk

1 tsp pure vanilla extract

Directions

1. Heat up oven to 350°F.

2. Prepare 12 regular-size cooking spray coated muffin cups.

3. Add cinnamon, salt, baking powder, baking soda, brown sugar, flaxseed and flour into a big bowl and whisk until combined.

4. Add banana and zucchini into the big bowl and stir until incorporated.

5. Add vanilla, lightly beaten eggs and milk into a small bowl and whisk until combined.

6. Add vanilla mixture into the flour mixture and stir to combine.

TIP: Be careful not to over mix.

7. Split batter between lightly coated muffin cups and transfer into the preheated oven.

8. Bake for 20-25 minutes until an inserted toothpick comes out clean.

9. Let muffins sit for 30 minutes on a wire rack, until wholly cooled.

10. Serve and enjoy or store in a well lidded container for up to 3 days.

Healthy Gingerbread Oatmeal

Preparation Time: 10 minutes

Cook Time: 20 minutes

Serves: 4 servings

Ingredients

1 cup steel cut oats

4 cups water

1/4 teaspoon coriander, ground

1 1/2 tablespoons cinnamon, ground

1/4 teaspoon ginger, ground

1/4 teaspoon cloves, ground

1/8 teaspoon nutmeg, ground

1/4 teaspoon allspice, ground

Honey, to taste

1/4 teaspoon cardamom, ground

Directions

1. Add water, spices and oats into pot over med-high heat.

2. Cook oats according to instructions on the package.

3. Serve and enjoy.

Poached Eggs and Curried Potatoes

Preparation Time: 10 minutes

Cook Time: 30 minutes

Serves: 4 servings

Ingredients

1" fresh ginger, peeled & grated

2 (about 2 pounds) russet potatoes, washed and cut into 3/4" cubes

1 tablespoon olive oil

2 minced garlic cloves

1 (15 ounce) can tomato sauce

2 tablespoons curry powder

1/2 bunch fresh cilantro, if desired

4 big eggs

Directions

1. Place potato cubes into a big pot over high heat, and add water until cubes are covered.

2. Bring mixture to boiling and keep boiling until fork-tender, for 5-6 minutes.

3. Drain off excess water and let potatoes sit until cooled.

4. Add olive oil, garlic and ginger into a big deep skillet over med-low heat and saute garlic mixture until aromatic and tenderized, for 1-2 minutes.

5. Add curry powder into the garlic mixture and saute until spices are toasted, for about a minute.

6. Stir in the tomato sauce, adjust heat to med-heat and cook sauce until heated through.

7. Check for seasoning and adjust salt if necessary.

8. Add the cooled potatoes into the sauce mixture and stir until coated with sauce.

9. Add few tbsps water if potato mixture seems dry.

10. Make 4 dips or holes in the potato mixture, and crack one big egg into each hole.

11. Cover skillet, and allow simmering.

12. Simmer potato mixture and eggs until cooked through, for 6-10 minutes.

13. Serve garnished with fresh chopped cilantro.

One-Sheet Tomatoes, Asparagus with Eggs

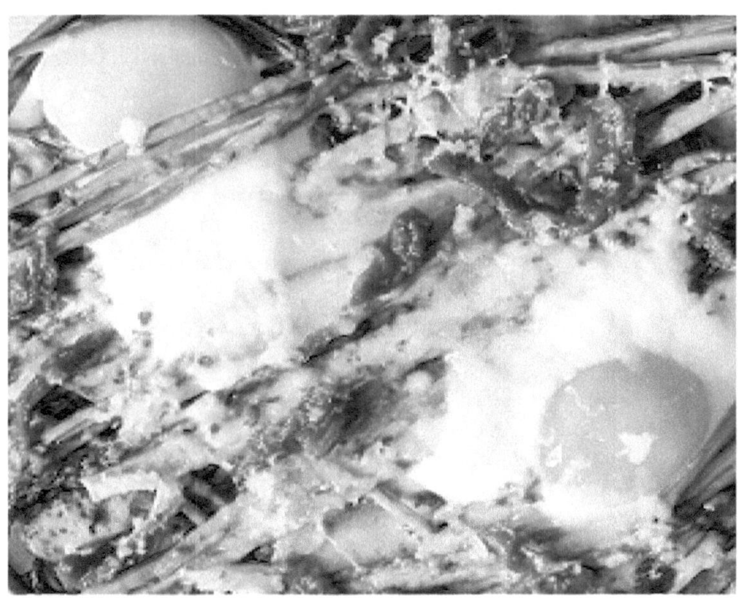

Preparation Time: 10 minutes

Cook Time: 20 minutes

Serves: 4 servings

Ingredients

1 pint cherry tomatoes

2 lbs. asparagus

2 tbsps avocado oil

4 eggs

Salt & pepper

2 tsps fresh thyme, chopped

Directions

1. Heat up oven to 400°F.

2. Prepare a rimmed nonstick cooking spray greased baking sheet.

3. Add cherry tomatoes and asparagus to the prepared baking in a single and even layer.

4. Dribble veggies with avocado oil and season with pepper, salt and thyme.

5. Transfer into the preheated oven and roast for 10-12 minutes, until the tomatoes are wrinkled and the asparagus are almost soft.

6. Take out baking sheet and crack eggs over veggies.

7. Season eggs with pepper and salt.

8. Place baking sheet into the oven and bake for 7-8 minutes until egg whites are set.

9. Split between four plates, serve and enjoy.

Orange Pineapple Smoothie

Preparation Time: 5 minutes

Cook Time: 0 minutes

Serves: 1 serving

Ingredients

1 (peeled) orange

1 ½ cups pineapple chunks, frozen

1/4 tsp ginger, ground

1 cup coconut water

1 tsp ground turmeric

1 tsp chia seeds

1/4 tsp black pepper, ground

Directions

1. Add every ingredient into a high speed electric blender.

2. Process mixture until a smooth consistency.

3. Serve smoothie, garnished with any remaining chia seeds.

Chia Turmeric Pudding

Preparation Time: 5 minutes

Cook Time: 0 minutes

Serves: 2-4 servings

Ingredients

1/3 cup chia seeds

1 1/2 cups unsweetened almond milk

1 teaspoon turmeric, ground

2 tablespoons honey

1/8 teaspoon cardamom, ground

1/2 teaspoon cinnamon

1/8 teaspoon cloves, ground

Directions

1. Add every ingredient into a bowl.

2. Mix until combined and let sit in a refrigerator for 8 hours or more until set.

3. Top with preferred nuts and fruits.

Peaches Almond Green Smoothie Bowl

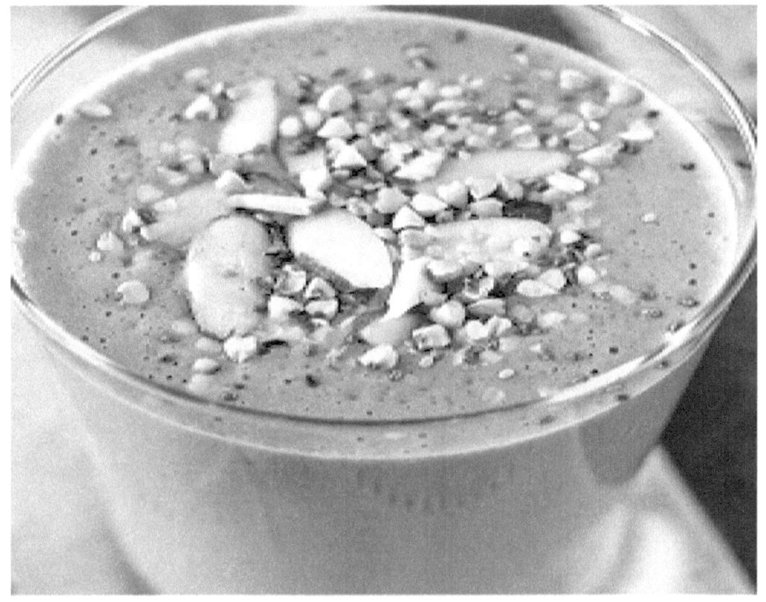

Preparation Time: 10 minutes

Cook Time: 0 minutes

Serves: 1 serving

Ingredients

½ cup sliced peaches, frozen

½ cup sliced banana, frozen

½ cup almond milk, unsweetened

1 cup fresh spinach

1½ tsps matcha tea powder

5 tbsps (split) slivered almonds

½ diced ripe kiwi

1 tsp honey

Directions

1. Add honey, matcha powder, 3 tbsps almonds, almond milk, spinach, peaches and banana into a high speed electric blender.

2. Process mixture until a fine and smooth consistency is reached.

3. Pour the blended smoothie into a bowl and add the remaining 2 tbsps slivered almonds and kiwi on top.

Almond Berry Smoothie Bowl

Preparation Time: 10 minutes

Cook Time: 0 minutes

Serves: 1 serving

Ingredients

½ cup sliced banana, frozen

1/3 cup raspberries, frozen

5 tbsps (split) almonds, sliced

½ cup almond milk, plain unsweetened

1/3 tsp cardamom, ground

¼ tsp cinnamon, ground

¼ cup blueberries

1/3 tsp vanilla extract

1 tbsp coconut flakes, unsweetened

Directions

1. Add vanilla, cardamom, cinnamon, 3 tbsps almonds, almond milk, banana and raspberries into a high speed electric blender.

2. Blend mixture until a smooth consistency is reached.

3. Pour the blended smoothie mixture into a bowl, topped with coconut, 2 tbsps almonds and blueberries.

Spinach Mushroom Frittata

Preparation Time: 15 minutes

Cook Time: 30 minutes

Serves: 4 servings

Ingredients

1/4 cup milk

6 eggs

1 (sliced thin) onion

1 cup cheddar cheese, grated

3 tbsps butter

4 ounces (sliced) white button mushrooms

Salt and pepper

2 cups baby spinach

Directions

1. Heat up oven to 350°F, with oven rack set in the center position.

2. Cover an 8" square baking dish with butter and let sit until needed.

3. Add milk and eggs into a big bowl, whisk until combined and season with pepper and salt.

4. Add butter into a big nonstick skillet over med-heat.

5. Add mushrooms and onions into the melted butter and brown.

6. Sprinkle with pepper and salt, add spinach, stir continuously and keep cooking for about a minute.

7. Add the browned mushrooms into the milk egg mixture and stir until combined.

8. Pour egg mixture into the prepared baking dish and transfer into the preheated oven.

9. Bake eggs until puffed and lightly browned, for about 25 minutes.

10. Slice frittata into 4 squares, and remove squares from the baking dish using a spatula.

11. Plate frittatas and dig in.

Cheesy Open Face Sandwich with Beet

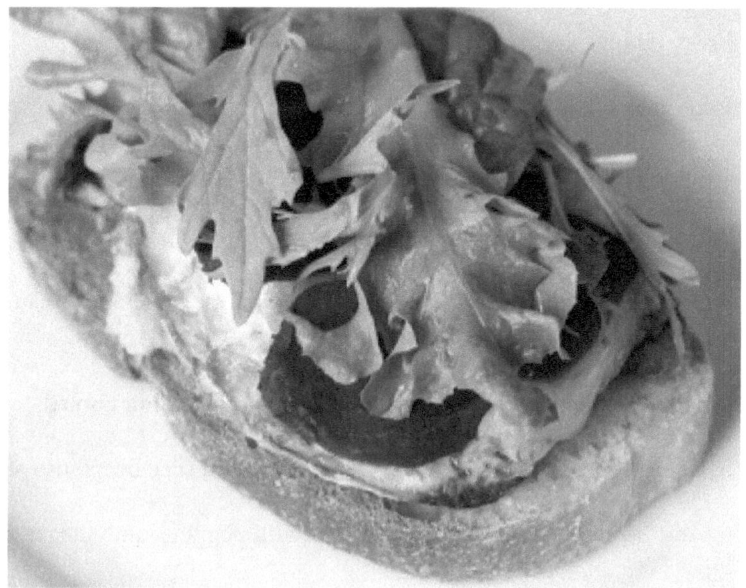

Preparation Time: 5 minutes

Cook Time: 15 minutes

Serves: 4 servings

Ingredients

1 tbsp canola oil

4 small (scrubbed) red beets

¼ tsp salt

1 tbsp white balsamic vinegar

4 oz. (at room temperature) soft goat cheese

Ground pepper

4 (1/2" thick) crusty whole-grain bread slices, lightly toasted

2 tbsps coconut milk

Garnish with

Fresh thyme

Directions

1. Fit a big saucepan with a steamer basket and place over med-high heat.

2. Add 1" of water into the saucepan.

3. Add beets into the saucepan, place lid over saucepan and steam beets, for 10-15 minutes.

4. Place steamed beets on cutting board and let sit until cooled.

5. Using a paper towel, scrub off beet skins, and slice beets into slices.

6. Add beet slices into a bowl and toss with pepper, salt, vinegar and canola oil.

7. Add coconut milk and goat cheese into a fairly big bowl and stir until combined.

8. Spread 2 tbsps of the milk cheese mixture on each toast slice.

9. Add some of the beets and garnish with fresh thyme.

10. Serve and enjoy.

Avocado Spinach Smoothie

Preparation Time: 5 minutes

Cook Time: 0 minutes

Serves: 1 serving

Ingredients

1 cup spinach, fresh

1 cup plain yogurt, nonfat

¼ avocado

1 banana, frozen

1 tsp maple syrup

2 tbsps water

Directions

1. Add maple syrup, water, avocado, banana, spinach and yogurt into a high speed electric blender.

2. Blend mixture until a smooth consistency is reached.

3. Serve and enjoy.

Almond Berry Chia Pudding

Preparation Time: 10 minutes

Cook Time: 0 minutes

Serves: 1 serving

Ingredients

2 tbsps chia seeds

½ cup coconut milk

1/3 tsp almond extract

2 tsps honey

1 tbsp (split) slivered almonds, toasted

½ cup (split) fresh blueberries

Directions

1. Add almond extract, honey, chia and coconut milk into a small bowl.

2. Stir chia mixture until combined.

3. Place lid over bowl and place in a refrigerator for 8 or more hours.

4. Stir refrigerated chia pudding to combine.

5. Scoop half of the pudding into another bowl, topped with half of the almonds and half of the blueberries.

6. Add the remaining half of the pudding into the bowl and top with the remaining almonds and blueberries.

Healthy Crepes

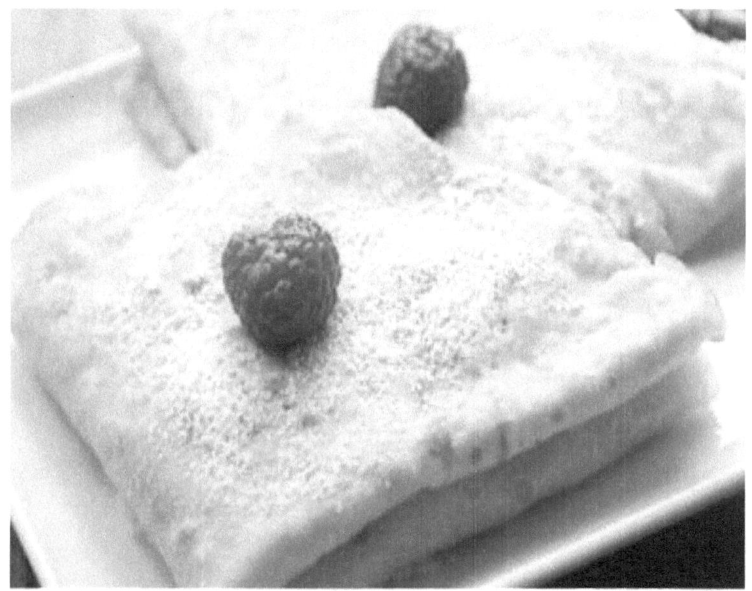

Preparation Time: 5 minutes

Cook Time: 20 minutes

Serves: 6 servings

Ingredients

1 tsp vanilla

2 eggs

1/2 cup water

1/2 cup almond milk

1-2 tbsps agave nectar

1/4 tsp salt

2 tbsps coconut oil + 1 tbsp

1 cup all purpose flour, gluten-free

Directions

1. Add 2 tbsps coconut oil into a small saucepan over low heat and melt.

2. Add agave nectar, salt, water, almond milk, vanilla and the eggs into a fairly big bowl and whisk until combined.

3. Add the flour into the egg mixture slowly and whisk until combined.

4. Slowly add in the melted oil into the flour mixture while slowly whisking continuously until combined.

5. Mix batter until a smooth consistency is reached.

6. Add coconut oil into a big frying pan over med-high heat.

7. Scoop about 1/3 cup of batter per crepe into the hot oil.

8. Swirl and tilt pan in rounded movements until pan surface is evenly coated.

9. Cook crepe until the base is light brown, for about 2 minutes; using a spatula flip the crepe and cook for about 2 more minutes.

10. Repeat process with the remaining batter, serve and enjoy.

Banana Peanut Butter Smoothie

Preparation Time: 5 minutes

Cook Time: 0 minutes

Serves: 1-2 servings

Ingredients

1 tablespoon peanut butter

1 banana

Maple syrup

10 ounces coconut milk

Directions

1. Add every ingredient into a high speed electric blender.

2. Blend until a smooth consistency is reached.

3. Serve and enjoy.

Peach Green Smoothie Bowl

Preparation Time: 10 minutes

Cook Time: 0 minutes

Serves: 1 serving

Ingredients

¾ cup almond milk, unsweetened

1 cup sliced peaches, frozen

¼ cup silken tofu

½ cup avocado, diced

1 tsp matcha tea powder

2 tsps honey

1 tbsp almonds, roughly chopped

¼ cup fresh blueberries

1 tsp hemp seeds

1 tbsp coconut flakes, unsweetened

Directions

1. Add matcha, honey, tofu, avocado, almond milk and peaches into a high speed electric blender.

2. Process mixture until a smooth consistency is reached.

3. Transfer blended smoothie mixture into a bowl, topped with hemp seeds and blueberries.

4. Serve and enjoy.

Almond Cranberry Granola Bars

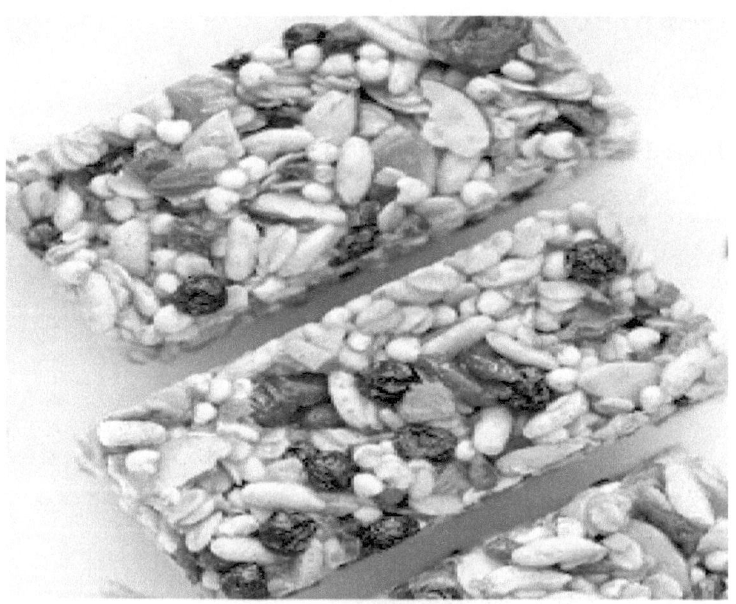

Preparation Time: 15 minutes

Cook Time: 35 minutes

Serves: 1 serving

Ingredients

1 cup crispy brown rice cereal

3 cups rolled oats, old-fashioned

½ cup (toasted & chopped) almonds

1 cup cranberries, dried

¼ tsp salt

½ cup (toasted & chopped) pecans

½ cup smooth almond butter

1/3 cup brown rice syrup

1 tsp vanilla extract

Directions

1. Heat up oven to 325°F.

2. Prepare a parchment paper lined 9x13" baking pan and grease lightly with cooking spray.

TIP: The parchment paper liner should hang over 2 sides of the baking pan.

3. Add salt, pecans, almonds, cranberries, rice cereal, and oats into a big bowl and combine.

4. Add vanilla, almond butter and brown rice syrup into a microwave-secure bowl and combine.

5. Place almond butter bowl into a microwave and heat for 30 seconds.

6. Add the almond butter mixture into the oats bowl and stir until incorporated and combined.

7. Pour mixture into the prepared baking pan; using a spatula, press oat mixture firmly into the baking pan.

8. Transfer baking pan into the preheated oven and bake for 30-35 minutes, until firm in the middle, and golden brown around the edges.

9. Let granola bar sit until cooled for 10 minutes before removing from the baking pan with the hanging parchment paper.

10. Place on a cutting board and slice into 24 granola bars.

11. Let sit for about 30 minutes, until completely cooled and separate.

Soy Berry Banana Smoothie

Preparation Time: 5 minutes

Cook Time: 0 minutes

Serves: 1-2 servings

Ingredients

5 ounces silken tofu

1 cup vanilla flavored soy milk

2 cups (sliced) fresh strawberries

1 (sliced into chunks) banana

2 teaspoons pure maple syrup

Directions

1. Add every ingredient into a high speed electric blender.

2. Blend until a smooth consistency is reached.

3. Serve and enjoy.

Avocado Berry Smoothie

Preparation Time: 5 minutes

Cook Time: 0 minutes

Serves: 1-2 servings

Ingredients

3/4 cup orange juice

1 (peeled & pitted) avocado

1/2 cup raspberries

3/4 cup raspberry juice

Directions

1. Add every ingredient into a high speed electric blender.

2. Blend until a smooth consistency is reached.

3. Serve and enjoy.

Delicious Tomato smoothie

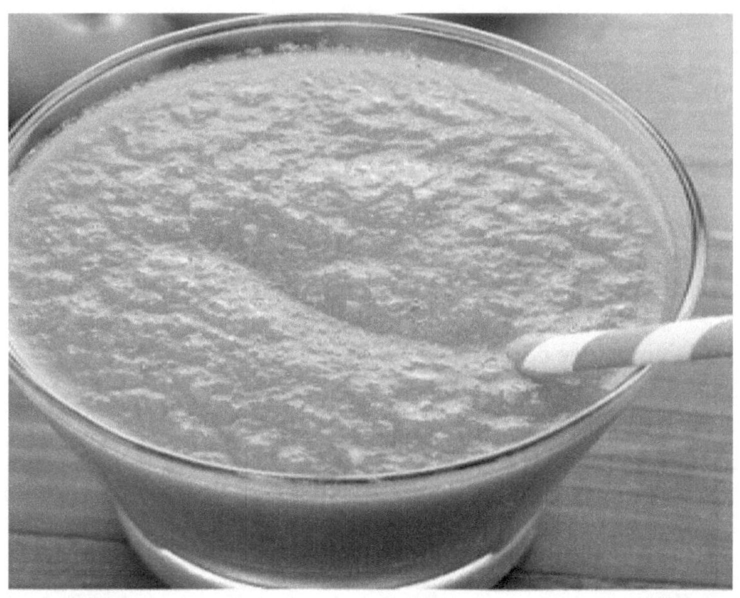

Preparation Time: 5 minutes

Cook Time: 0 minutes

Serves: 1-2 servings

Ingredients

1/2 cup tomato juice

2 cups tomatoes

1/2 cup carrots

1/4 cup apple juice

Hot sauce

1/4 cup celery

2 cups ice

Directions

1. Add every ingredient into a high speed electric blender.

2. Blend until a smooth consistency is reached.

3. Serve and enjoy.

Fiber-Rich Kale Smoothie

Preparation Time: 5 minutes

Cook Time: 0 minutes

Serves: 1-2 servings

Ingredients

2 bananas

4-5 kale leaves (soak in water until softened)

A few slices cucumber

1 cup blueberries

Directions

1. Add every ingredient into a high speed electric blender.

2. Blend until a smooth consistency is reached.

3. Serve and enjoy.

Lemon Papaya Mango Smoothie

Preparation Time: 5 minutes

Cook Time: 0 minutes

Serves: 1-2 servings

Ingredients

1/4 teaspoon almond extract

3 tablespoons pure maple syrup

2 tablespoons freshly squeezed lemon juice

2 cups plain yogurt

1 (peeled & seeded) papaya

1 (peeled & pitted) mango

Directions

1. Add every ingredient into a high speed electric blender.

2. Blend until a smooth consistency is reached.

3. Serve and enjoy.

Lunch

Walnuts with Roasted Grapes & Brussels Sprouts

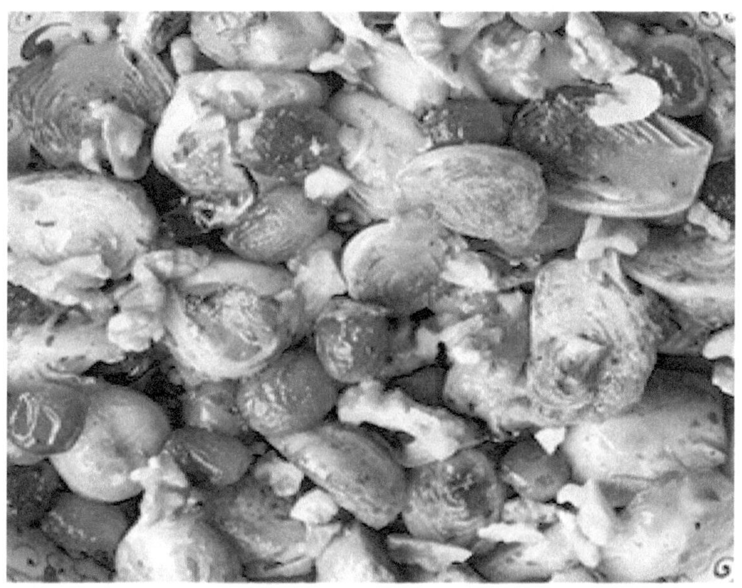

Preparation Time: 10 minutes

Cook Time: 20 minutes

Serves: 8 servings

Ingredients

24 oz. grapes

8 cups (halved or quartered) Brussels sprouts

4 tbsps fresh thyme

2 tbsps avocado oil

2 tsps brown rice vinegar

Coarse salt and freshly ground pepper

1/2 cup (toasted and roughly chopped) walnuts

Directions

1. Heat up oven to 450°F.

2. Add grapes and Brussels sprouts to a very large rimmed baking sheet or two rimmed baking sheets.

3. Add thyme and avocado oil to sprouts mixture and toss until coated.

4. Season sprouts mixture with pepper and salt.

5. Place baking sheet into the preheated oven and roast for about 20 minutes until softened and caramelized.

6. Dribble 1 tsp brown rice vinegar over each baking tray or 2 tsp for 1 large baking tray.

7. Use a wooden spoon; scrape up bits of caramelized sprouts and grapes.

8. Sprinkle walnuts over roasted sprouts and grapes

Vegetable Burgers with Quinoa and Beet

Preparation Time: 10 minutes

Cook Time: 10 minutes

Serves: 8 servings

Ingredients (Burgers)

5 tbsps flax meal, split

1 1/2 cups eggplant, chopped

4 cups beets, shredded

6 tbsps warm water

1 cup rolled oats, gluten-free

1 cup quinoa, cooked

1/2 cup hummus

2 minced garlic cloves

Avocado oil

Salt and pepper, to taste

Serve with

Hummus

Greens

Gluten-free buns

Directions

1. Add fresh eggplants into a steaming basket and steam for about 5 minutes until fork-soft.

2. Add steamed eggplants into a food process and puree on high until a smooth consistency is reached.

3. Pour pureed eggplants into a bowl and let sit until needed.

4. Add water, and 2 tbsps flax meal, stir well and let sit for later use.

5. Add garlic, the remaining 3 tbsps flax meal, oats, quinoa and beets into a food processor.

6. Process mixture until combined and pour into the bowl.

7. Add hummus, the pureed eggplant and flax and warm water mixture into the bowl with the processed quinoa mixture.

8. Mix until dough is dense and can be shaped into patties.

9. Season dough with pepper and salt.

NOTE: If dough appears too wet, let sit for 10-15 more minutes before adding more flax meals to soak up some of the moisture.

10. Prepare a parchment paper lined baking sheet and form 8 patties from dough.

11. Place patties on the prepared baking sheet and refrigerate for 60 minutes or more until chilled.

12. Add oil into a skillet over med-heat.

13. Place burgers in hot oil and sear for about 3-4 minutes on each side.

14. Place browned burger on a wire rack to cool and repeat process with the remaining patties.

15. Serve burgers with buns, topped with humus and greens.

Stuffed Peppers with Sweet Potato and Ground Chicken

Preparation Time: 10 minutes

Cook Time: 50 minutes

Serves: 4 servings

Ingredients

2 cup ground chicken

1 tablespoon avocado oil

½ cup diced onions

2 minced garlic cloves

½ cup tomato sauce

1 2/3 cup (diced) sweet potato

Salt and pepper

Crushed red pepper, if desired

Fresh chopped cilantro

2 (cut in half) big bell peppers

Directions

1. Heat up oven to 350°F.

2. Add avocado oil into a skillet over med-high heat.

3. Add garlic and ground chicken into the hot oil and cook until meat is no longer pink, for about 10 minutes. Stir every now and then to break meat apart.

4. Add onions into the skillet and cook until golden brown.

5. Add sweet potato into the skillet, place lid over skillet and cook for about 8 minutes until softened.

TIP: Stir mixture from time to time.

6. Add pepper, salt, ground chili pepper and tomato sauce into the skillet.

TIP: You can add a little bit of water into the mixture to thin out.

7. Lay halved bell peppers on a pre-greased baking dish with the hole-side up.

8. Fill each halves of bell pepper with the sweet potato and ground chicken mixture.

9. Place baking dish in the oven and roast until peppers are tender and cooked through for about 30 minutes, without covering.

10. Take peppers out of the oven and serve, garnished with cilantro.

Snap Pea Turkey Stir-Fry

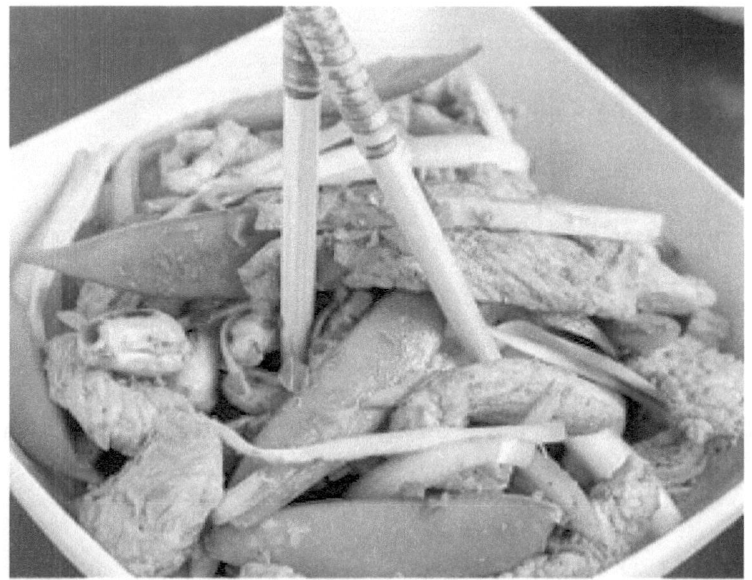

Preparation Time: 10 minutes

Cook Time: 10 minutes

Serves: 4 servings

Ingredients

1 (sliced thin) bunch scallions

2 tbsps olive oil

1 (sliced thin) red bell pepper

2 minced garlic cloves

1¼ cups (sliced thin) turkey breast, boneless skinless

2½ cups snap peas

3 tbsps soy sauce

Salt & freshly ground black pepper

2 tsps Sriracha, if desired

2 tbsps rice vinegar

3 tbsps fresh parsley, chopped

2 tbsps sesame seeds

Directions

1. Add oil into a big saute pan over med-heat.

2. Add garlic and scallions into the hot oil and saute for a minute until aromatic.

3. Add snap peas and bell pepper into the garlic mixture and saute for 2-3 minutes until just soft.

4. Add turkey slices into the pan and cook for 4-5 minutes, until veggies are softened and turkey is fully cooked and golden.

5. Add sesame seeds, sriracha (if desired), rice vinegar and soy sauce into the mixture, toss until combined and simmer for 1-2 minutes.

6. Add parsley and stir until incorporated.

7. Serve garnished with sesame seeds and any remaining parsley.

Turmeric Quinoa Bowls

Preparation Time: 10 minutes

Cook Time: 30 minutes

Serves: 4 servings

Ingredients

1 (15 ounces) can chickpeas, drain & rinsed

7 (sliced into strips) yellow potatoes, small

1 teaspoon paprika

2 teaspoons turmeric

1/4 cup quinoa

1 tablespoon avocado oil

2 kale leaves

Salt/ground pepper

1 (sliced) avocado

1/2 tablespoon olive oil

Directions

1. Heat up oven to 350°F.

2. Lay potato strips flat on one side of a baking sheet.

3. Season with 1 teaspoon of turmeric and dribble avocado oil over potatoes.

4. Sprinkle pepper and salt over potatoes to taste.

5. Transfer baking sheet into the preheated oven and roast for 5 minutes.

6. In the meantime, add 1 teaspoon paprika and the chickpeas into a bowl and mix until wholly coated.

7. Add coated chickpeas into the empty side of the baking sheet and return into the oven.

8. Roast potatoes and chickpeas until the potatoes are just tenderized, for about 25 minutes.

9. Add 1/2 cup water and quinoa into a pot over med-heat.

10. Cook quinoa according to directions on the package.

11. Add pepper, salt and 1 teaspoon turmeric into the cooked quinoa and mix until combined.

12. Let quinoa sit until cool.

13. Rub olive oil into washed kale leaves, and split kale leaves between 4 serving bowls.

14. Split avocado slices between the serving bowls and top with the roasted potatoes, chickpeas and quinoa.

Quick and Delicious Fried Rice with Pineapple

Preparation Time: 10 minutes

Cook Time: 20 minutes

Serves: 4 servings

Ingredients

1 tbsp sesame oil

3 tbsps soy sauce

1/4 tsp white pepper

1/2 tsp ginger powder

2 minced garlic cloves

2 tbsps olive oil

2 (peeled & grated) carrots

1 diced onion

1/2 cup peas, frozen

1/2 cup corn, frozen

2 cups fresh pineapple, diced

3 cups brown rice, cooked

2 sliced green onions

1/2 cup ham, diced

Directions

1. Add white pepper, ginger powder, sesame oil and soy sauce into a small bowl, whisk until combined and let sit until needed.

2. Add olive oil into a big skillet over med-high heat.

3. Add onion and garlic into the skillet and stir cook for about 3-4 minutes until onions are translucent.

4. Add peas, corn and carrots into the skillet and stir cook for about 3-4 minutes, until the veggies are softened.

5. Add soy sauce mixture, green onions, ham, pineapple and rice into skillet and stir until combined.

6. Cook for about 2 minutes until warmed through.

7. Serve at once.

Parchment Wrapped Lemon Ginger Salmon

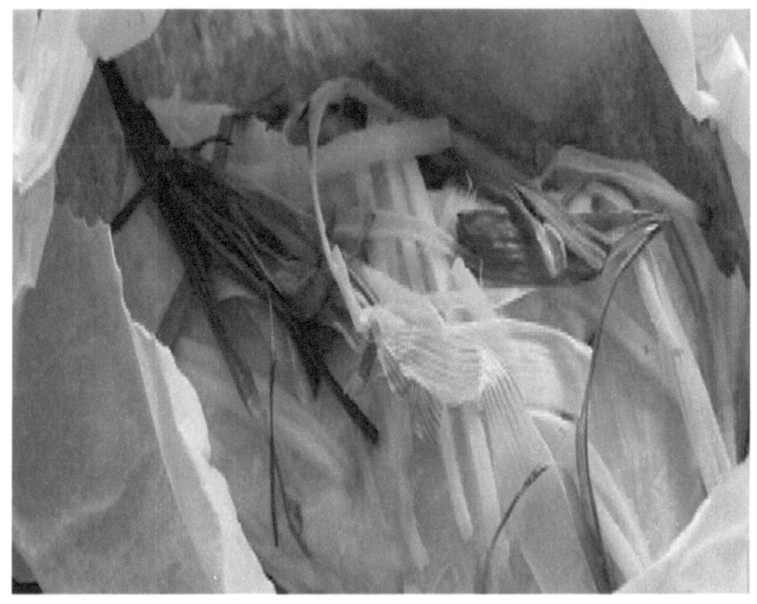

Preparation Time: 10 minutes

Cook Time: 20 minutes

Serves: 4 servings

Ingredients

2 tbsps soy sauce

1 tsp sesame oil

1 tsp garlic powder

2 tbsps fresh ginger, grated

1 pinch red-pepper flakes

2 tbsps pure maple syrup

1 (halved and sliced thin) red onion

2 (halved lengthways and sliced thin) large zucchini

4 (6-oz.) salmon fillets, skinless

1 (divided) lemon, juiced

4 tsps sesame seeds

Directions

1. Heat up oven to 350°F.

2. Prepared 4 parchment pieces (about 15x17").

3. Fold each parchment piece in half until a crease is formed, unfold and let parchment sit until needed.

4. Add red pepper flakes, maple syrup, garlic powder, ginger, soy sauce and sesame oil into a small bowl and whisk until combined.

5. Add an even layer of zucchini, topped with red onion and lemon juice into one side of each parchment piece.

6. Repeat process until all parchment pieces are evenly packed with veggies and drizzle with equal amounts of lemon juice.

7. Top each parchment pack with a salmon fillet, and liberally cover salmon with the soy sauce and sesame oil mixture.

8. Top each parchment pack with 1 tsp sesame seeds.

9. Fold empty parchment side over veggies and salmon, tuck parchment edges until parchment wrap is well sealed.

10. Place salmon parchment wraps on a baking sheet and transfer into the preheated oven.

11. Bake salmon wraps for 16-18 minutes, until well cooked.

12. Place vegetables and salmon onto serving platter, serve at once and enjoy.

Tzaztziki Sauced Chicken Burgers

Preparation Time: 35 minutes

Cook Time: 35 minutes

Serves: 4 servings

Ingredients (Burgers)

1 minced sweet onion

1 tbsp olive oil

1 egg

2 minced garlic cloves

½ tsp oregano, dried

½ cup fresh parsley, chopped

1 lb. ground chicken

¼ tsp red-pepper flakes

Salt & freshly ground black pepper

¾ cup bread crumbs

Sauce

½ diced English cucumber

1 cup Greek yogurt

2 tbsps lime juice

1 tbsp olive oil

Salt & freshly ground black pepper

1 pinch garlic powder

¼ cup fresh cilantro, chopped

Toppings

½ sliced red onion

4 hamburger buns, whole-wheat

2 sliced tomatoes

8 Boston lettuce leaves

Directions

1. Add olive oil into a small skillet over med-heat.

2. Add onions into the hot oil and cook for 3-4 minutes until soft.

3. Add garlic into the oil mixture and saute for a minute more.

4. Set skillet aside until cooled to room temperature.

5. Add ground chicken, red pepper flakes, oregano, parsley, egg and the cooled garlic mixture into a fairly big bowl and combine.

6. Add bread crumbs into the mixture, stir until combined and season with pepper and salt.

7. Heat up oven to 375°F.

8. Form chicken burger mixture into 4 even patties.

9. Place a big oven-secure skillet over med-high heat and cover liberally with nonstick cooking spray.

10. Sear burgers in the skillet for 4-5 minutes on each side.

11. Place skillet with burgers into the preheated oven and cook for 15-17 more minutes, until chicken burgers are fully cooked.

12. Add garlic powder, lime juice, olive oil, cucumber and yogurt into a fairly big bowl and combine for the sauce.

13. Sprinkle pepper and salt over sauce.

14. Stir in cilantro into the sauce until incorporated.

15. Place each cooked burger on the underneath half of a bun, topped with 2 tomato slices, 2 lettuce leaves, about 1/4 cup tzaztziki sauce and the other bun half.

16. Serve at once and enjoy.

Ratatouille with Zucchini and Bell Pepper

Preparation Time: 35 minutes

Cook Time: 55 minutes

Serves: 4 servings

Ingredients

2 smashed garlic cloves

5 tbsps olive oil

1 cup tomato puree

2 sprigs oregano

1 (sliced thickly) medium red onion

1 (sliced thickly) small eggplant

2 (sliced thickly) medium zucchini

2 (sliced thickly) medium summer squash

3 (sliced thickly) medium tomatoes

2 (sides cut off & halved) small red bell peppers

Salt & freshly ground black pepper

2 tbsps thyme leaves

Directions

1. Heat up oven to 375°F.

2. Place 1 (9" square) baking dish on a baking sheet.

3. Add olive oil into a small pot over med-low heat.

4. Add garlic into the pot and cook for a minute until aromatic.

5. Take pot off heat, stir in oregano into the pot and let sit for 15 minutes until flavors are infused.

6. Get rid of the oregano and garlic.

7. Dribble 2 tbsps olive oil into the bottom of the baking dish.

8. Add and spread 1/4 cup tomato puree into the bottom of the baking dish.

9. Lay tomato, pepper, zucchini, summer squash, onion and eggplant into the baking dish until tightly packed.

10. Brush veggie layers with the remaining tomato puree and dribble with the remaining olive oil until wholly covered.

11. Season with pepper, salt and thyme.

12. Place baking sheet into the preheated oven and roast for 25-30 minutes, until the edges and surface is just brown, and softened.

13. Let sit for 5-10 minutes until cooled before you serve.

Dinner

Spaghetti Squash Stuffed with Chickpea and kale

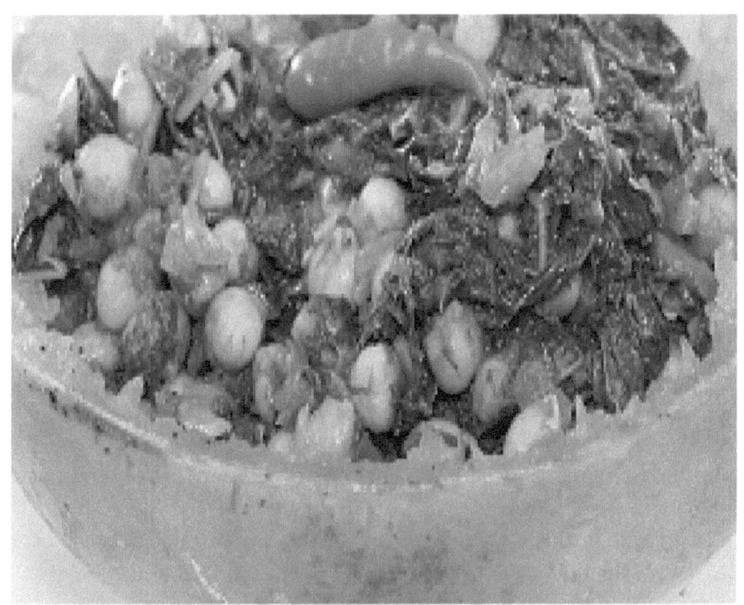

Preparation Time: 15 minutes

Cook Time: 40 minutes

Serves: 2 servings

Ingredients

4-5 (wash & remove large stems) handfuls kale

1 (halved and scoop out strings and seeds) spaghetti squash

1 cup (drained & rinsed) chickpeas

2 minced garlic cloves

Avocado oil

1/4 cup slivered almonds

Sea salt and pepper

Directions

1. Heat up oven to 400°F.

2. Lightly coat the cavity of the spaghetti squash halves with avocado oil and season with pepper and salt.

3. Transfer seasoned squash halves onto a baking sheet with the cavity side down.

4. Transfer baking sheet into the preheated oven and bake for 40 minutes.

5. In the meantime, add olive oil into a fairly big skillet over med-heat.

6. Add minced garlic into the hot oil and saute for 1 minute.

7. Add slivered almonds into the skillet with the garlic and saute until the almonds are just toasted and the garlic is aromatic, for some minutes.

8. Add kale into the skillet mixture, season with salt, stir until combined and distributed, and saute until kale wilts

9. Add the chickpeas into the skillet mixture and mix until evenly distributed.

10. Scoop kale mixture into the baked spaghetti squash halves until filled and serve.

One-Sheet Zucchini and Lime Herb Salmon

Preparation Time: 15 minutes

Cook Time: 20 minutes

Serves: 4 servings

Ingredients (zucchini)

2 tbsps avocado oil

4 (chopped) zucchini

Kosher salt and freshly ground black pepper, to taste

Salmon

2 tbsps lime juice, freshly squeezed

2 tbsps packed brown sugar

2 minced garlic cloves

1 tbsp Dijon mustard

1/2 tsp oregano, dried

1/2 tsp dill, dried

1/4 tsp rosemary, dried

1/4 tsp thyme, dried

4 (5-oz.) salmon fillets

Kosher salt and freshly ground black pepper, to taste

2 tbsps fresh cilantro, chopped

Directions

1. Heat up oven to 400°F.

2. Prepare a lightly greased baking sheet.

3. Add rosemary, thyme, oregano, dill, garlic, Dijon, lime juice and brown sugar into a small bowl and whisk until combined.

4. Sprinkle rosemary mixture with pepper and salt as necessary and let sit until needed.

5. Add zucchini onto the baking sheet in one layer, season with pepper and salt and dribble with avocado oil.

6. Add salmon fillets onto the baking sheet in one layer and brush with the rosemary mixture.

7. Place baking sheet into the oven and cook for about 16-18 minutes, until salmon flakes easily, using a fork.

8. Serve at once and garnish with fresh chopped cilantro.

Cauli-Rice and Salmon Bowl

Preparation Time: 10 minutes

Cook Time: 35 minutes

Serves: 2 servings

Ingredients

10-12 (chopped in half) Brussels sprouts

2 organic salmon fillets

½ (riced) head cauliflower

1 (washed & shredded) bunch kale

1 tsp curry powder

3 tbsps olive oil

Himalayan salt

Marinade

1 tsp Dijon mustard

¼ cup tamari sauce

1 tsp honey, if desired

1 tsp sesame oil

1 tbsp sesame seeds

Directions

1. Heat up oven to 350°F.

2. Add chopped Brussels sprouts on a parchment paper lined baking sheet.

3. Cover sprouts with 1 tbsp oil until evenly coated.

4. Season sprouts with salt and place baking sheet in the preheated oven.

5. Roast for 20 minutes.

6. In the meantime, add every marinade ingredient into a bowl and whisk to combine.

7. Take out sprouts from the oven; add the fish fillets to the baking sheet.

8. Evenly cover fish fillets with the marinade and place in the oven.

9. Bake until fish is well cooked, for 13-15 more minutes.

10. Add 1 tbsp oil into a skillet over med-high heat.

11. Add kale in hot oil and saute for 2-3 minutes until kale wilts.

12. Take kale off pan and let sit until needed.

13. Add the remaining oil into the same skillet and add the cauliflower rice.

14. Season cauliflower rice with salt, and 1 tsp curry powder.

15. Saute cauliflower rice for 2-3 minutes until well cooked.

16. Split Brussels sprouts and salmon between 2 serving bowls, top with cauli-rice and kale.

17. Serve and enjoy.

Veggie Coconut Curry with Chickpea

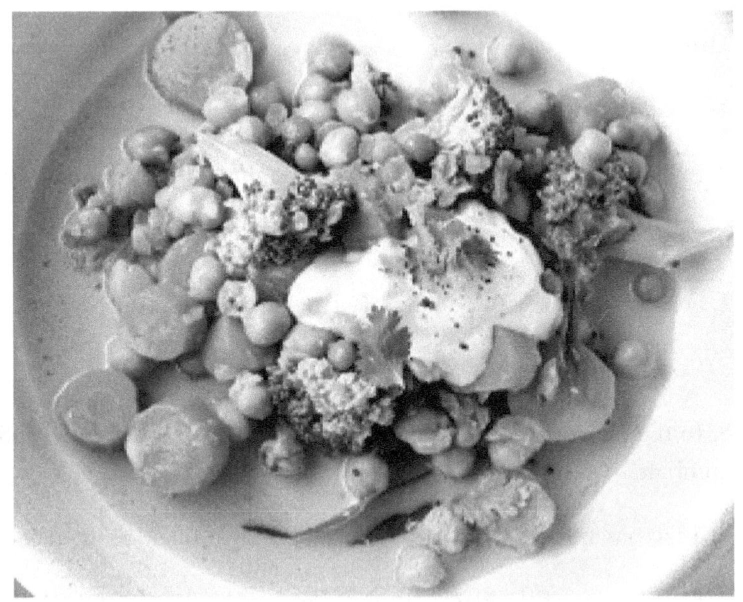

Preparation Time: 10 minutes

Cook Time: 20 minutes

Serves: 4 servings

Ingredients

1 (sliced thin) red onion

1 tbsp olive oil

1 tbsp minced fresh ginger

1 (sliced thin) red bell pepper

1 (cut into bite sized florets) small head cauliflower

3 minced garlic cloves

1 tsp coriander, ground

2 tsps chile powder

1 (14-oz.) can coconut milk

3 tbsps red curry paste

1 (28-oz.) can cooked chickpeas

1 (halved) lemon

Salt & freshly ground black pepper

1½ cups frozen peas

4 (sliced thin) scallions

¼ cup fresh parsley, chopped

Directions

1. Add olive oil into a big pot over med-heat.

2. Add bell pepper and onion into the hot oil and saute for about 4-5 minutes, until just soft.

3. Add garlic and ginger into the mixture and saute for a minute until aromatic.

4. Add cauliflower into the mixture and toss well until combined.

5. Add the red curry paste, coriander and chile powder into the mixture, stir until combined and cook for a minute until the whole mixture is slightly darkened.

6. Add coconut milk into the pot, stir until incorporated and bring to simmering over med-low heat.

7. Place lid over pot and keep simmering for 8-10 minutes, until the cauliflower is softened.

8. Uncover pot, add lemon juice into the mixture and stir until evenly distributed.

9. Add pepper, salt, peas and chickpeas into the curry and bring mixture to simmering.

10. Serve and enjoy, garnished with 1 tbsp scallion and 1 tbsp parsley.

Indian Saag Paneer

Preparation Time: 10 minutes

Cook Time: 16 minutes

Serves: 4 servings

Ingredients

¼ tsp turmeric, ground

8 oz. (sliced into 1/2" cubes) paneer cheese

1 (chopped finely) small onion

2 tbsps (split) canola oil

1 minced garlic clove

1 (chopped finely) jalapeño pepper

2 tsps garam masala

1 tbsp fresh ginger, minced

20 oz. (thawed and chopped finely) frozen spinach

1 tsp ground cumin

2 cups plain yogurt, low-fat

¾ tsp salt

Directions

1. Add turmeric and paneer cheese into a fairly big bowl and toss until covered.

2. Add 1 tbsp canola oil into a big nonstick skillet over med-heat.

3. Add the turmeric coated cheese into the hot oil and cook for about 5 minutes, until browned on each sides.

TIP: Flip cheese once.

4. Plate browned paneer cheese and add the remaining 1 tbsp canola oil into the skillet.

5. Add jalapeno and onion into the hot oil and stir cook for 7-8 minutes until golden brown.

TIP: Add 2 tbsps water per time while cooking to moisten skillet if it seems too dry.

6. Add cumin, garam masala, ginger and garlic into the skillet and stir cook for about 30 seconds until aromatic.

7. Add salt and spinach into the skillet and stir cook for about 3 minutes until heated through.

8. Take skillet off heat, add the paneer cheese and yogurt and stir until distributed.

9. Serve alone or over rice.

Potato Curry Soup with Roasted Cauliflower

Preparation Time: 15 minutes

Cook Time: 1 hour 10 minutes

Serves: 8 (1 1/2 cup) servings

Ingredients

2 tsps cumin, ground

2 tsps coriander, ground

1½ tsps turmeric, ground

1½ tsps cinnamon, ground

¾ tsp ground pepper

1¼ tsps salt

6 cups cauliflower florets

1/3 tsp cayenne pepper

1 (chopped) large onion

2 tbsps (split) olive oil

3 minced big garlic cloves

1 cup carrot, diced

1 minced jalapeno pepper

1½ tsps fresh ginger, grated

4 cups veggie broth, low-sodium

1 (14 oz.) can tomato sauce, no-salt-added

3 cups sweet potatoes (peeled & diced into ½-inch cubes)

3 cups russet potatoes (peeled & diced into ½-inch cubes)

2 tsps lemon zest

1 (14 oz.) can coconut milk

2 tbsps lemon juice

Directions

1. Heat up oven to 450°F.

2. Add cayenne, pepper, salt, turmeric, cinnamon, cumin and coriander into a small bowl and combine.

3. Add 1 tbsp oil and cauliflower florets into a bug bowl and toss to coat.

4. Sprinkle 1 tbsps seasoning mixture over cauliflower and toss until wholly covered.

5. Add the seasoned cauli-florets into a rimmed baking sheet in one layer.

6. Place baking sheet in the preheated oven and roast for about 15-20 minutes, until cauliflower edges are browned.

7. Let roasted cauliflower sit to cool.

8. In the meantime, add 1 tbsp oil into a big pot over med-high heat.

9. Add carrot and onion into the hot oil and stir cook for about 3-4 minutes, until just brown.

10. Adjust heat to med-heat and keep cooking for 3-4 minutes until onion is tenderized, stirring frequently.

11. Add the remaining seasoning mixture, chile, ginger and garlic into the pot and stir cook for a minute more.

12. Add the tomato sauce into the pot, stir until distributed and simmer for a minute.

13. Add lemon juice, lemon zest, sweet potatoes, russet potatoes and veggie broth into the pot and stir until combined.

14. Place lid over pot and bring soup mixture to boiling over high heat.

15. Adjust heat until a gentle simmer is maintained, cover pot partially and stir cook for about 35-40 minutes, until veggies are softened.

16. Add roasted cauliflower and coconut milk into the soup and stir until evenly distributed.

17. Bring soup to simmering and serve garnished with parsley and chiles, if desired.

Spiced lentils with Greens and Roasted Root Veggies

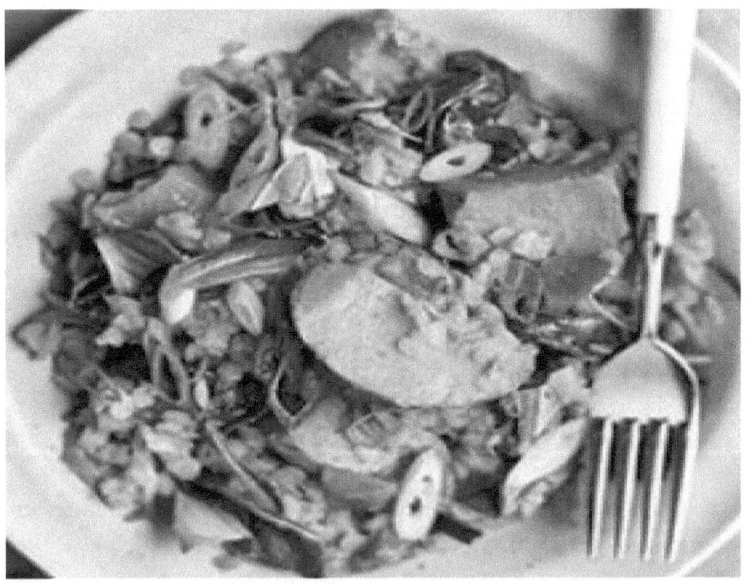

Preparation Time: 15 minutes

Cook Time: 45 minutes

Serves: 2 servings

Ingredients (Lentils)

½ cup black beluga lentils

1½ cups water

½ tsp coriander, ground

1 tsp garlic powder

¼ tsp allspice, ground

½ tsp cumin, ground

2 tbsps lime juice

¼ tsp kosher salt

1 tsp olive oil

Veggies

1 smashed garlic clove

1 tbsp olive oil

2 cups kale, chopped

1½ cups root vegetables, roasted

1/3 tsp ground pepper

1 tsp coriander, ground

2 tbsps plain yogurt, low-fat

Pinch of kosher salt

Garnish with

Fresh chopped cilantro

Directions

1. Add 1/4 tsp salt, cumin, 1/2 tsp coriander, garlic powder, lentils and water into a fairly big pot and combine.

2. Bring mixture to boiling, lower heat, place lid over pot and simmer for 25-30 minutes until softened.

3. Take off lid and simmer for about 5 more minutes until cooking juices evaporates slightly.

4. Drain and stir in 1 tsp oil and lime juice until evenly distributed.

5. Add oil into a big skillet over med-heat.

6. Add the garlic into the hot oil and cook for 1-2 minutes until aromatic.

7. Add the roasted veggies into the skillet and stir cook for 2-4 minutes until heated through.

8. Add the kale into the skillet mixture and cook for 2-3 minutes until kale wilts slightly.

9. Add salt, pepper and coriander into the skillet mixture and stir to combine.

10. Plate lentils, topped with veggies and yogurt.

11. Garnish each serving with fresh chopped cilantro.

Tomato, Chickpeas with Braised Cauliflower

Preparation Time: 15 minutes

Cook Time: 1 hour 15 minutes

Serves: 4 servings

Ingredients

1 (stems & leaves removed) large whole cauliflower

2 tbsps avocado oil

1 (15-oz.) can {drained & rinsed} chickpeas

1 (28-oz.) can tomato, crushed

1/4 cup nutritional yeast (if desired)

5-6 kale, ribs removed and chopped

2 tsps oregano, dried

3 minced garlic cloves

Salt and pepper, as needed

Directions

1. Heat up oven to 350°F.

2. Add oil into Dutch oven over med-high heat.

3. Add whole cauliflower into the hot oil and sear for about 10 minutes, rotating continuously until cauliflower outside is brown.

4. Take out cauliflower and place on a platter to cool.

5. Add pepper, salt, oregano, garlic, nutritional yeast, kale, chickpeas and tomato into the Dutch oven and cook for 3-4 minutes.

6. Add cauliflower into the tomato mixture and scoop mixture over cauliflower until coated.

7. Cover the Dutch oven and transfer into the preheated oven.

8. Bake cauliflower for about 60 minutes, until a toothpick inserted can go in easily.

9. Take out of the oven, let sit until cooled and slice.

10. Serve cauliflower slices with the tomato mixture and dig in.

Chickpeas, Veggies with Turmeric Rice Bowl

Preparation Time: 25 minutes

Cook Time: 50 minutes

Serves: 2 servings

Ingredients (Rice)

½ cup brown basmati rice

1¼ cups water

1 tsp olive oil

¼ cup raisins

½ tsp turmeric, ground

1 tsp garlic powder

¼ tsp black pepper, ground

¼ tsp cinnamon, ground

Kosher salt

Chickpeas and Veggies

1 (15 oz.) can {rinsed & pat dried} chickpeas

2 tbsps coconut oil

1 cup root vegetables, roasted

1 tsp garam masala

¼ tsp kosher salt

1 tsp honey

2 tbsps lime juice

¼ tsp ground pepper

2 tbsps plain yogurt, low-fat

Garnish with

Fresh chopped cilantro

Fresh chopped parsley

Fresh chopped mint

Directions

1. Add cinnamon, salt, pepper, garlic powder, olive oil, raisins, rice and water into a small saucepan over med-heat and combine.

2. Bring mixture to boiling, place lid over saucepan, adjust heat to low and simmer rice mixture for 35-40 minutes, until cooking juices evaporates.

3. Take off heat and let sit until cooled for 10 minutes without uncovering.

4. In the meantime, add coconut oil into a fairly big skillet over med-heat.

5. Add chickpeas into the hot oil and stir cook for 3-5 minutes until crispy.

6. Add garam masala into the skillet, stir until incorporated and cook for about a minute until aromatic.

7. Add pepper, salt, honey and roasted root veggies into the skillet.

8. Stir cook for about 2-4 minutes until warmed through.

9. Add the lime juice into the skillet mixture and stir until incorporated.

10. Serve the veggie mixture over cooked rice.

11. Top rice and veggies with low-fat plain yogurt and garnish with herbs.

Cranberries, Brussels Sprouts with Balsamic Turkey

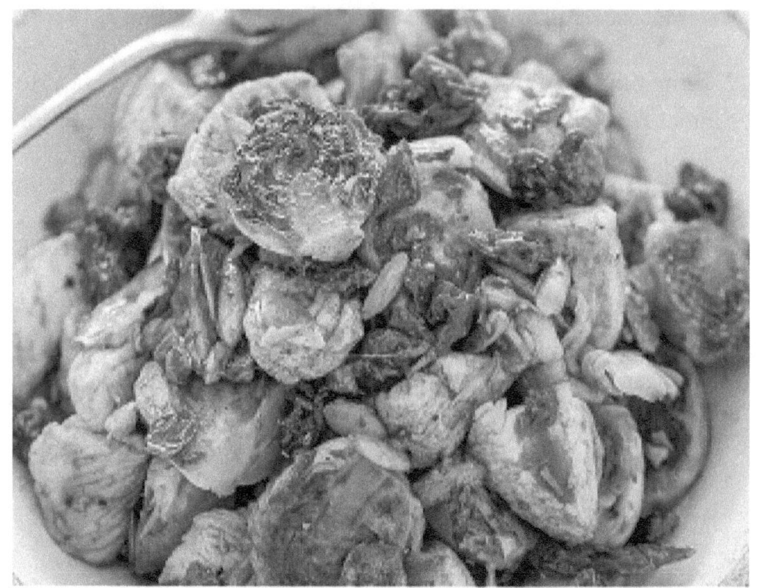

Preparation Time: 5 minutes

Cook Time: 15 minutes

Serves: 4 servings

Ingredients

15-20 (trimmed & halved lengthways) Brussels sprouts

3 tbsps (split) olive oil

1 (peeled & diced small) large shallot

1 1/4 lbs. (diced into bite-sized pieces) turkey breast, boneless skinless

1/4 cup balsamic vinegar

Salt and pepper

1/2 cup (dry, not oil-packed) sun-dried tomatoes

2 tbsps pure maple syrup

1/2 cup roasted pumpkin seeds

1/2 cup cranberries, dried

Directions

1. Add 2 tbsps olive oil into a big skillet over med-high heat.

2. Add the Brussels sprouts with the cut side down into the skillet and cook until slightly golden brown and seared, for about 4-5 minutes.

3. Flip Brussels sprouts over and push to a side of the skillet.

4. Add the remaining 1 tbsp olive oil into the empty side of the skillet and add the shallots and turkey.

5. Sprinkle with pepper and salt and cook until turkey until well cooked, for about 4-5 minutes, flipping and stirring turkey every now and then.

6. Add maple syrup and balsamic vinegar into the turkey mixture and stir until distributed.

7. Adjust heat to med-low, and simmer until Brussels sprouts are crisp-soft, and turkey is well cooked, for about 2-3 minutes.

8. Add pumpkin seeds, cranberries and sun-dried tomatoes into the skillet and stir until evenly distributed.

9. Serve at once and enjoy, can be store in a well lidded container and refrigerated for up to 5 days.

Fennel, Turmeric Roasted Turkey

Preparation Time: 15 minutes

Cook Time: 45 minutes

Serves: 4-6 servings

Ingredients

1/2 cup dry white wine

1/2 cup olive oil

1 lemon, juiced

1/2 cup orange juice

3 tablespoons brown sugar

2 tablespoons yellow mustard

3/4 tablespoon turmeric spice, ground

1 tablespoon garlic powder

1 teaspoon sweet paprika

1 teaspoon coriander, ground

1 (cored & sliced) large fennel bulb

Salt & Pepper

6 pieces turkey breasts, bone in, skin on (pat dried)

1 (sliced into 1/2 moons) large sweet onion

1 lemon, sliced thin (if desired)

2 (unpeeled & sliced) oranges

Directions

1. Add brown sugar, mustard, lemon juice, orange juice, white wine and olive oil into a big bowl.

2. Mix until combined.

3. Add pepper, salt, paprika, coriander, garlic powder and turmeric into a small bowl and combine.

4. Add 1/2 of the turmeric mixture into the lemon juice marinade and stir until combined.

5. Liberally season turkey pieces with the remaining turmeric mixture until wholly covered.

TIP: Add turmeric spice mix under turkey skin by carefully lifting turkey skin,

6. Add every other ingredient and the seasoned turkey into the bowl with the lemon juice marinade until evenly covered.

7. Place lid over bowl and transfer into a refrigerator for 1-2 hours.

8. Heat up oven to 475°F.

9. Place marinade, turkey and every other ingredient from the bowl into a big baking pan in a single layer.

TIP: Turkey should be place with the skin facing up.

10. Transfer baking pan into the preheated oven and roast until turkey is nicely browned and well cooked, for 40-45 minutes.

11. Serve and enjoy.

Spicy Chickpea Cakes

Preparation Time: 10 minutes

Cook Time: 10 minutes

Serves: 4 servings

Ingredients

2 garlic cloves

1 small onion

1/4 cup (coarsely chopped) fresh parsley

1 can chickpeas, rinsed and drained

1-2 tsps sea salt

2 tbsps potato starch

1 tsp turmeric powder

Freshly ground black pepper

2 tbsps + 3tbsps chickpea flour

1/2–1 tsp cayenne pepper, if desired

Olive oil

Directions

1. Add olive oil into a big cast iron skillet over med-heat.

2. Add garlic and onion into the hot oil and fry until golden.

TIP: Make sure you don't burn the garlic mixture.

3. Take skillet off heat and let sit until cooled.

4. Add chickpeas into a food processor and process until a just textured paste-like consistency is reached.

TIP: Scrape food processor insides every now and then.

5. Add in cayenne pepper, turmeric, pepper, salt, garlic and onion into the food processor.

6. Process until combined, switch off the processor, add in chopped parsley and stir until incorporated.

7. Sprinkle a few tbsps of chickpea flour onto a big plate.

8. Scoop chickpea mixture into cleans and form golf-sized balls.

9. Press each ball gently until patties are made.

10. Place chickpea patties into the plate until evenly and lightly coated with chickpea flour.

11. Dust off any excess flour sticking to the patties.

12. Place the same skillet over med-heat.

13. Add more olive oil into the skillet and add patties into the hot oil.

14. Cook until nicely browned, for 2-3 minutes per side.

15. Serve turmeric cakes with veggies or salad and enjoy.

Avocado Dipping Sauce with Roasted Sweet Potatoes

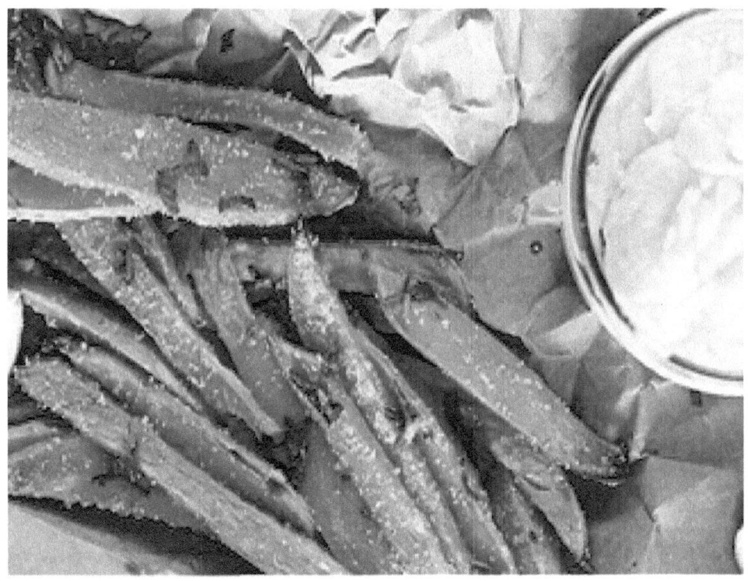

Preparation Time: 10 minutes

Cook Time: 45 minutes

Serves: 4 servings

Ingredients

1 tsp olive oil

2 (washed & cut into 1/2" square cubes) large sweet potatoes

1 (halved & pitted) avocado

1/2 tsp sea salt

1 lemon, juiced

1 (peeled & chopped) big garlic clove

2 tbsp olive oil

2-4 tbsp water

Directions

1. Heat up oven to 400°F.

2. Evenly spread potato cubes on a baking pan.

3. Dribble olive oil over sweet potato cubes.

4. Toss and flip sweet potato cubes until each cube is lightly coated.

5. Re-spread sweet potato cubes in one layer and season with 1/4 tsp sea salt.

6. Transfer baking pan into the preheated oven and bake until sweet potatoes are lightly browned, for 40-45 minutes.

7. Add avocado into a high speed electric blender with 1/4 tsp salt, lemon juice, and garlic.

8. Blend avocado mixture until a creamy and smooth consistency is reached.

9. Add water in a slow and steady stream and keep blending until combined.

10. Add olive oil in a slow and steady stream until incorporated while blending.

11. Blend until combined and a creamy texture forms.

12. Serve roasted sweet potato cubes with avocado dipping sauce.

Beverage

Lime Turmeric Tea

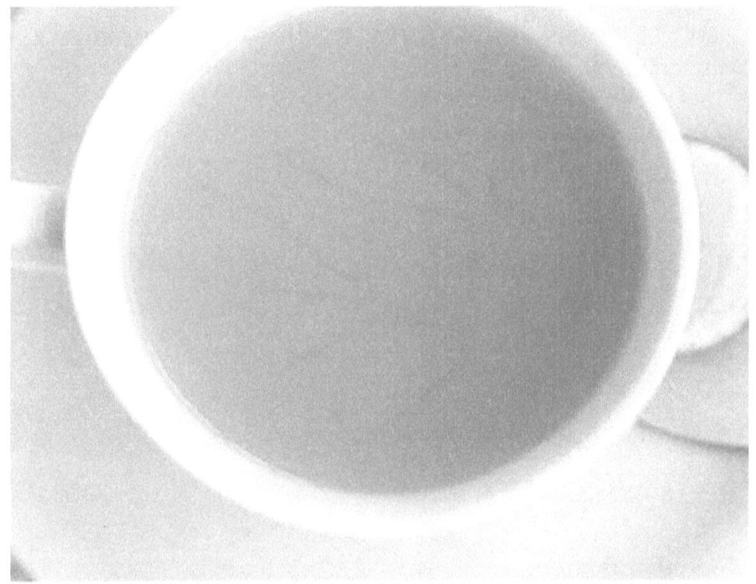

Preparation Time: 5 minutes

Cook Time: 10 minutes

Serves: 1 qt. servings

Ingredients

1/2 tsp turmeric

3 1/2 cups water

1 lime, peeled without pith

3 tbsps maple syrup

1 pinch cayenne

2 tbsps lime juice

Directions

1. Add every ingredient into a saucepan over med-heat.

2. Bring mixture to boiling, take off heat and cover.

3. Let tea mixture sit until flavors are infused and tea is cooled to room temperature.

4. Strain tea, reheat and serve.

Healthy Hot Chocolate

Preparation Time: 5 minutes

Cook Time: 0 minutes

Serves: 1 serving

Ingredients

1/2 tsp cinnamon

1 tbsp raw cacao powder

1/2 tsp turmeric, dried

1/4 tsp ginger, dried

1 pinch cardamom, if desired

1 pinch cayenne pepper

1 pinch sea salt

1/2 tsp rice malt syrup

1/2 cup warmed coconut milk

Freshly ground black pepper

1/2 cup water

Directions

1. Add pepper, sea salt, dried spices and raw cacao powder into a regular mug.

2. Add rice malt syrup and boiling water into the cacao powder mixture until the mug is halfway filled.

3. Stir until mixture dissolves.

4. Add warmed coconut milk into the mug and stir until evenly distributed.

5. Serve and enjoy.

Delicious Blueberry Smoothie

Preparation Time: 5 minutes

Cook Time: 0 minutes

Serves: 1 serving

Ingredients

1 banana, frozen

2 spinach handfuls

1 tablespoon almond butter

1/2 cup raspberries, frozen

1/8-1/4 teaspoon cayenne pepper

1/4 teaspoon cinnamon

1/2 cup water

1 teaspoon maca powder, if desired

1/2 cup coconut milk, unsweetened

Directions

1. Add every ingredient into a high speed electric blender.

2. Process mixture until a smooth consistency is reached.

3. Pour into a bowl and serve at once.

Delicious Turmeric Latte

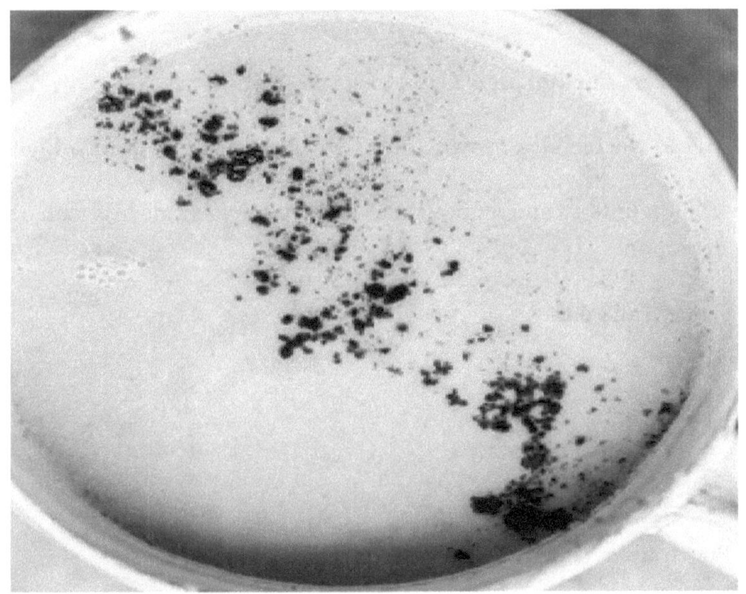

Preparation Time: 5 minutes

Cook Time: 5 minutes

Serves: 1 serving

Ingredients

1 tbsp fresh turmeric, grated

1 cup almond milk, unsweetened

1 tsp fresh ginger, grated

2 tsps honey

1 pinch of ground pepper

Garnish with, if desired

Ground cinnamon

Directions

1. Add pepper, ginger, honey,turmeric and almond milk into a high speed electric blender.

2. Process mixture until a smooth consistency is reached,

3. Pour the blended mixture into a small saucepan over med-high heat.

4. Cook until steaming; pour into a regular mug garnished with a sprinkle of cinnamon.

5. Serve and enjoy.

Therapeutic Chamomile Tonic with Herbs

Preparation Time: 20 minutes

Cook Time: 0 minutes

Serves: 4 (1 cup) servings

Ingredients

6 bags chamomile tea

4 cups boiling water

4 slices lime

2 tsps fresh ginger, grated

2 lightly bruised rosemary sprigs

2-4 tsps honey

Directions

1. Add rosemary, honey, lime slices, ginger, chamomile tea bags and boiling water into a big oven-safe bowl.

2. Let sit until flavors are infused for 20 minutes, stirring every now and then.

3. Use a fine mesh sieve to strain tonic and press tea bags to remove as much liquid as likely,

4. Serve and enjoy.

Delicious Green Tea Latte

Preparation Time: 5 minutes

Cook Time: 5 minutes

Serves: 1 serving

Ingredients

1 tsp matcha tea powder

¼ cup boiling water

1 tsp honey

1 cup low-fat milk

Directions

1. Add matcha powder and boiling water into a high speed electric blender.

2. Blend mixture until a foamy consistency is reached.

3. Add honey and milk into a pot over med-heat.

4. Heat honey mixture until just boiling and whisk thoroughly until a frothy consistency is reached.

5. Pour milk into a regular mug and add the blended tea.

6. Stir, serve and enjoy.

Blueberry antioxidant smoothie

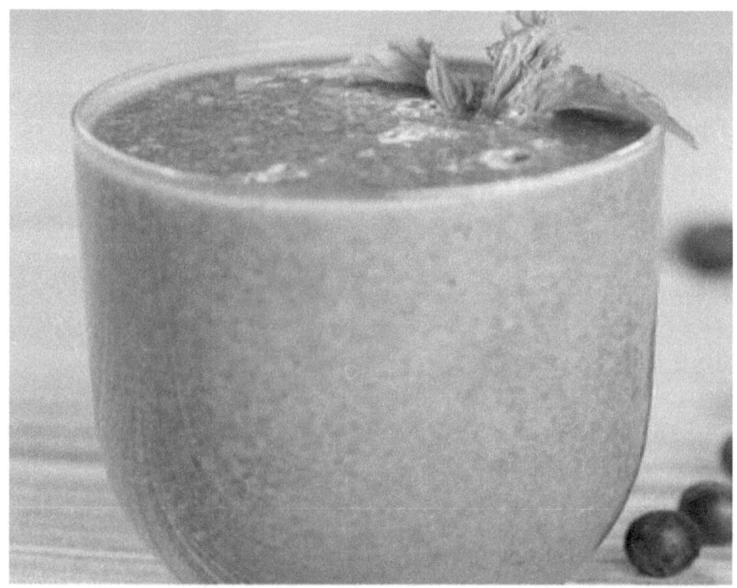

Preparation Time: 5 minutes

Cook Time: 0 minutes

Serves: 1-2 servings

Ingredients

1/2 cup plain yogurt

1 cup blueberries

1 tablespoon condensed milk

1 cup milk, low-fat

Directions

1. Add every ingredient into a high speed electric blender.

2. Blend until a smooth consistency is reached.

3. Serve and enjoy.

Iced Pineapple Banana Smoothie

Preparation Time: 5 minutes

Cook Time: 0 minutes

Serves: 1-2 servings

Ingredients

4 fluid ounces cream of coconut

2 bananas

3 cups ice, crushed

1 (8 ounces) can (with juice) pineapple chunks

Greek yogurt

Directions

1. Add every ingredient into a high speed electric blender.

2. Blend until a smooth consistency is reached.

3. Serve, garnished with coconut flakes and enjoy.

Whey Protein Power Smoothie

Preparation Time: 5 minutes

Cook Time: 0 minutes

Serves: 1-2 servings

Ingredients

1 cup 2% milk

1 cup yogurt

1 scoop whey protein powder

1 banana

1/2 cup ice

Directions

1. Add every ingredient into a high speed electric blender.

2. Blend until a smooth consistency is reached.

3. Serve and enjoy.

Salad

Grilled Turkey Wrap with Kale Caesar Salad

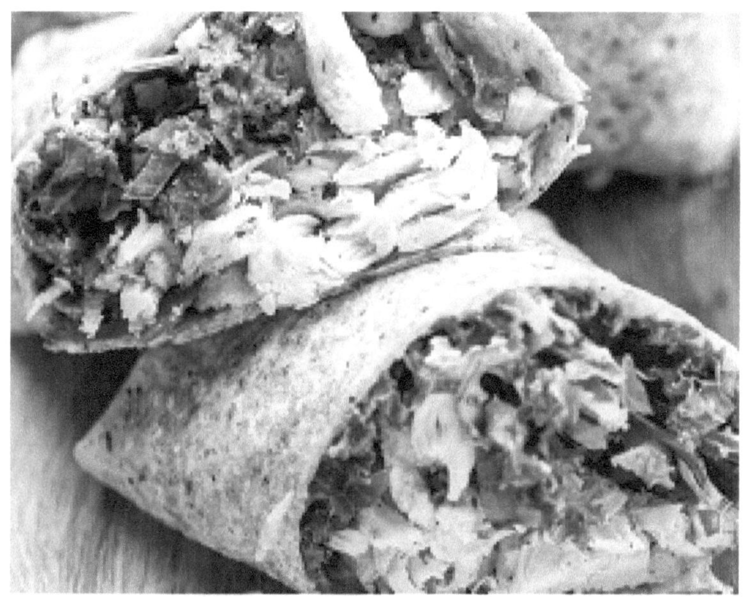

Preparation Time: 10 minutes

Cook Time: 0 minutes

Serves: 2 servings

Ingredients

6 cups (cut into bite sized pieces) curly kale

8 oz. (sliced thin) grilled turkey

3/4 cup Parmesan cheese, finely shredded

1 cup (quartered) cherry tomatoes

1 minced garlic clove

½ (cooked for about a minute) coddled egg

1 tsp honey

1/2 tsp Dijon mustard

1/8 cup avocado oil

1/8 cup fresh lime juice

2 large tortillas

Salt and freshly ground black pepper

Directions

1. Add avocado oil, lime juice, honey, mustard, minced garlic and half of a coddled egg into a bowl and mix until combined.

2. Whisk mixture until a dressing consistency is reached.

3. Sprinkle with pepper and salt.

4. Add 1/4 cup parmesan, cherry tomatoes, grilled turkey and kale into the dressing and toss until coated.

5. Spread out 2 tortillas, and top with the salad evenly and sprinkle each tortilla with 1/4 cup parmesan.

6. Roll tortilla wraps, slice in half, serve at once and enjoy.

Orange Bulgur Sweet Potato Salad

Preparation Time: 10 minutes

Cook Time: 50 minutes

Serves: 4-6 servings

Ingredients

1 tbsp avocado oil

2 (peeled & diced) medium sweet potatoes

Coarse salt and freshly ground black pepper

2 tsps honey, if desired

¼ cup olive oil

1¼ cups bulgur wheat

2 tbsps lime juice

¼ cup orange juice, freshly squeezed

1 minced, small clove garlic

1 tbsp red wine vinegar

Black pepper to taste

½ tsp salt

½ cup mint, finely chopped

1 cup parsley, finely chopped

2 tbsps orange zest

¼ cup red onion, finely chopped if desired)

Directions

1. Heat up oven to 425°F.

2. Add pepper, a liberal pinch of coarse salt, honey, avocado oil into a bowl, combine and toss with the sweet potatoes until coated.

3. Transfer coated sweet potatoes onto a parchment paper lined baking.

4. Place baking sheet into the preheated oven and roast until gently caramelized and completely softened, for 35-40 minutes.

TIP: Stir sweet potatoes halfway while roasting.

5. In the meantime, add 3 1/2 cups into a pot over med-heat and bring to boiling.

6. Add bulgur into the boiling water, adjust heat to low heat, stir every now and then, and simmer bulgur for 8 minutes.

7. Take off the pot from heat, place lid over pot and let bulgur stand for 10 minutes until cooled.

8. Drain off any surplus water and use a fork to fluff bulgur.

9. Add pepper, salt, garlic, red wine vinegar, lime juice, orange juice and olive oil into a bowl and whisk until combined.

10. Add orange zest, red onion, mint, parsley, the cooked bulgur and the sweet potatoes into a big mixing bowl.

11. Add the orange juice vinegar dressing into the sweet potato bowl and toss well until combined.

12. Check for seasoning and adjust as necessary.

Easy Grilled Eggplant Salad

Preparation Time: 15 minutes

Cook Time: 10 minutes

Serves: 4 servings

Ingredients

1 (sliced into rounds) large red onion

1 (cut into 1" thick slices) Italian eggplant

1 (halves, pitted, peeled & chopped) avocado

Avocado oil

1 tsp Dijon mustard

1 tbsp red wine vinegar

Maple syrup

1 tbsp oregano leaves, coarsely chopped

Salt

Olive oil

1 lime, zested

Freshly ground black pepper

Garnish with

Fresh chopped cilantro

Directions

1. Cover red onions and eggplant with avocado oil.

2. Place oil coated red onions and eggplants on the grill and spread.

3. Grill onions until just charred, and the eggplants are tenderized.

4. Take off onions and eggplants from the grill and place on a cutting board until slightly cooled.

5. Coarsely chop the cooled eggplants and onions and transfer into a serving bowl.

6. Add chopped avocado into the serving bowl.

7. Add oregano, Dijon, and red wine vinegar into a small bowl and whisk until combined.

8. Add olive oil and maple syrup into the oregano mixture and blend until emulsified

9. Sprinkle pepper and salt over mixture.

10. Toss grilled eggplants salad with dressing until combined.

11. Serve, garnished with cilantro and lime zest.

Quick and Easy Greek Salad

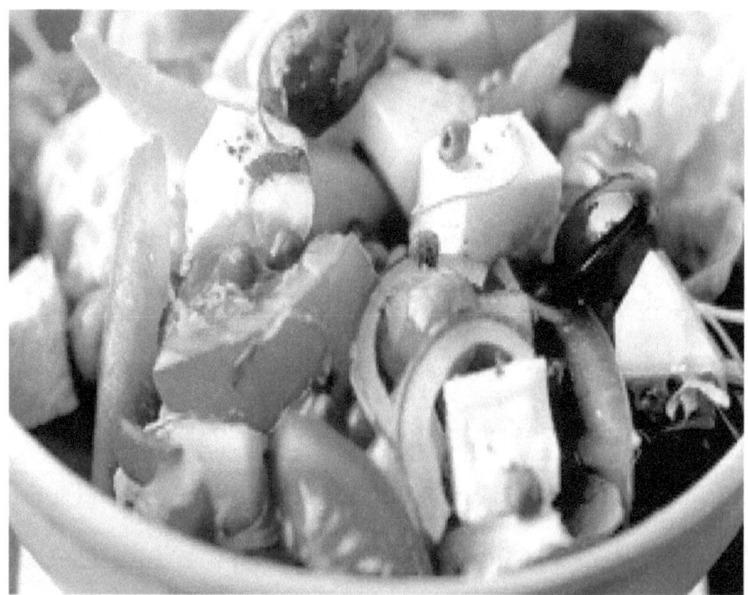

Preparation Time: 10 minutes

Cook Time: 10 minutes

Serves: 8 servings

Ingredients

1/2 cup black olives

4 (cut into spears) small cucumbers

1 lb. (sliced) Greek feta cheese

1 (sliced thin) red onion

Sea salt and freshly ground pepper

Olive oil

Garnish with

Fresh chopped parsley.

Directions

1. Add cheese, onion, olives, cucumbers and tomatoes into a plate.

2. Dribble olive oil over salad and sprinkle with pepper and salt.

3. Serve garnished with fresh chopped cilantro.

Spinach Tuna Salad

Preparation Time: 10 minutes

Cook Time: 0 minutes

Serves: 1 serving

Ingredients

1½ tbsps lime juice

1½ tbsps tahini

1 (5-oz.) can {drained} chunk light tuna in water

1½ tbsps water

2 tbsps feta cheese

4 (pitted & chopped) Kalamata olives

2 cups baby spinach

2 tbsps cilantro

1 (peeled & sliced) medium orange

Directions

1. Add water, lime juice and tahini into a bowl and whisk until combined.

2. Add cilantro, feta, olives and tuna into the bowl and stir until evenly distributed.

3. Serve 2 cups of spinach into a bowl and top with the lime tuna salad.

4. Add orange slices on the side; serve and enjoy.

Maple Walnuts, Cheese with Red Cabbage Salad

Preparation Time: 10 minutes

Cook Time: 10 minutes

Serves: 8 servings

Ingredients

¼ cup canola oil + 1 tbsp

1 tbsp blue cheese, crumbled

1 tbsp Dijon mustard

3 tbsps red-wine vinegar

¼ tsp freshly ground pepper

¼ tsp salt

1 cup walnuts

1 tsp butter

¼ tsp freshly ground pepper

¼ tsp salt

8 cups red cabbage, sliced very thin

3 tbsps pure maple syrup

1/3 cup blue cheese, crumbled

2 (sliced thin) scallions

Directions

1. Add pepper, salt, mustard, 1/4 cup oil and 1 tbsp blue cheese into a high speed electric blender or food processor.

2. Blend dressing mixture until a smooth and creamy consistency is reached.

3. Position a parchment paper piece near the stove.

4. Add butter and 1 tbsp canola oil into a fairly big skillet over med-heat.

5. Add walnuts into the butter mixture and stir cook for about 2 minutes.

6. Add maple syrup, pepper and salt into the skillet and stir cook for 3-5 more minutes until the nuts are just caramelized and well covered.

7. Add maple coated walnut with cooking juices onto the parchment paper, and separate walnuts while still warm.

8. Let walnuts sit to cool for 5 minutes or more.

9. Add scallions and cabbage into a big bowl and toss with the blended dressing.

10. Serve and top with maple coated walnuts and blue cheese.

Beets, Edamame with Green Salad

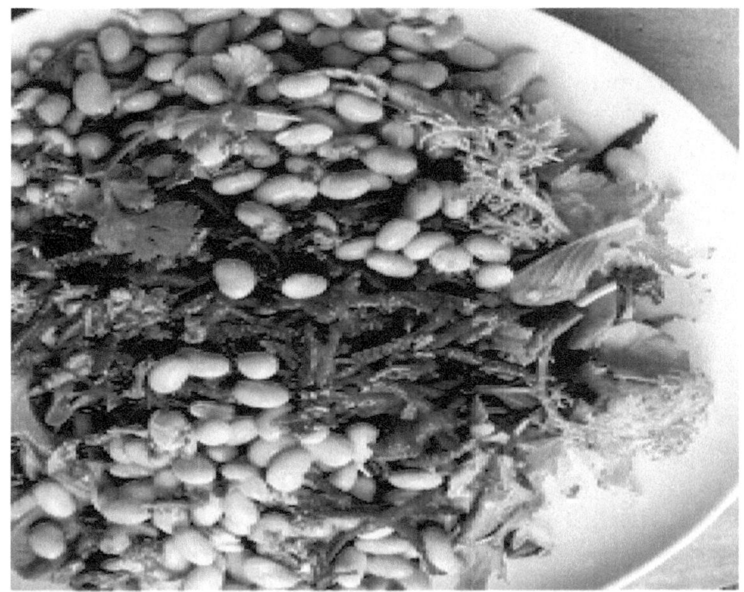

Preparation Time: 10 minutes

Cook Time: 0 minutes

Serves: 1 serving

Ingredients

1 cup (thawed) shelled edamame

2 cups mixed salad greens

1 tbsp red wine vinegar + 1½ tsps

½ (peeled & shredded) medium raw beet

2 tsps canola oil

1 tbsp fresh cilantro, chopped

Freshly ground pepper

Directions

1. Place beet, edamame and greens on a big platter.

2. Add pepper, salt, oil, cilantro and vinegar into a small bowl and whisk until combined.

3. Drizzle vinaigrette over green salad mixture.

4. Serve and enjoy.

Bacon with Watercress Berry Salad

Preparation Time: 20 minutes

Cook Time: 10 minutes

Serves: 4 servings

Ingredients (Bacon)

¼ cup port

8 oz. (cut crosswise into 14" thick strips) thick-cut bacon

1 tbsp honey

¼ cup red wine

1½ tsps 5-spice powder

2 peeled garlic cloves

Salad

2 tbsps canola oil

1 (sliced thin) medium shallot

1 tsp honey

2 tbsps lime juice

Pinch of sea salt

¼ tsp 5-spice powder

3 (cut into 1/4" wedges) firm ripe peaches

¾ cup fresh blueberries

½ (leaves separated & sliced into 1" strips) small head radicchio

4 cups (tough stems trimmed) watercress

Directions

1. Place a big skillet over med-heat.

2. Add the bacon into the hot skillet and stir cook for 3-5 minutes, until browned and crisp.

3. Using a slotted spoon, place browned bacon into a plate lined with paper towel.

4. Get rid of the bacon fat, place pan over heat adjust to high heat.

5. Add 1 1/2 tsp 5-spice powder, garlic cloves, honey, wine and port into the skillet.

6. Bring mixture to boiling.

7. Add the browned bacon into the skillet mixture and stir cook for about 2-3 minutes, until the sauce coats the bacon and is almost wholly evaporated.

8. Take skillet off heat.

9. Add salt, 5-spice powder, honey, oil, vinegar and the shallot into a big bow, and combine.

10. Add the blueberries into the bowl, crush with the back end of a spatula and stir until distributed.

11. Add radicchio, watercress and peaches into the salad bowl and toss until combined.

12. Plate salad, topped with the glazed bacon.

Cheesy Pistachios Roasted Beet Salad

Preparation Time: 15 minutes

Cook Time: 1 hour 15 minutes

Serves: 4 servings

Ingredients

4 cups chard, chopped

2 (trimmed) medium beets

1 tbsp sherry vinegar

8 Pixie tangerines

½ tsp (split) kosher salt

¼ tsp Dijon mustard

6 tsps (split) canola oil

Ground pepper, as needed

¼ cup toasted unsalted pistachios (roughly chopped)

¼ cup feta cheese, crumbled

Directions

1. Heat up oven to 375°F.

2. Scrub beets thoroughly, transfer moist beets into foil and wrap.

3. Transfer foil-wrapped beet into a small baking pan and transfer into the preheated oven and bake for 60-75 minutes, until and inserted knife tip enters into beet easily.

4. Let beet sit until cooled for 15 minutes before unwrapping.

5. Unwrap beets and set aside for 10 more minutes until wholly cooled.

6. Rub off beet skins using a kitchen towel, and trim the ends off.

7. Cut beets into slices and let sit until needed.

8. Rinse chard, drain and let sit until needed.

TIP: Chard should still be slightly moist.

9. Grate 1/2 tsp tangerine zest from a tangerine.

10. Cut off tangerine ends; peel off tangerine with the white pith.

11. Slice tangerine into segments and let sit until needed.

12. Add a liberal amount of ground pepper, 1/4 tsp salt, mustard, vinegar and tangerine zest into a fairly big bowl and combine.

13. Add 4 tsps canola oil into the zest mixture and whisk until evenly distributed.

14. Add the beet slices into the zest dressing mixture and toss until coated.

15. Let the beet mixture sit for 15 minutes.

16. Add 2 tsps canola oil into a big nonstick skillet over med-heat.

17. Add 1/4 tsp salt and the greens into the hot oil, gently stir and cook for 2-3 minutes until just wilted.

18. Split greens between 4 salad platters, topped with pistachios, cheese, tangerine and the beets.

19. Dribble any remaining dressing over salad, serve and enjoy.

Ginger Vinaigrette with Delicious Spinach Salad

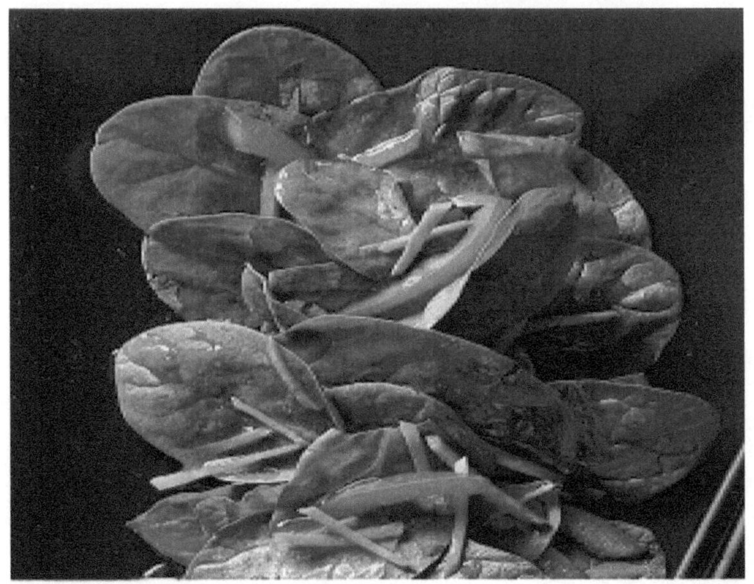

Preparation Time: 15 minutes

Cook Time: 0 minutes

Serves: 4 servings

Ingredients

3 tbsps olive oil

3 tbsps onion, minced

1½ tbsps fresh ginger, finely grated

2 tbsps distilled white vinegar

1 tbsp soy sauce, reduced-sodium

1 tbsp ketchup

¼ tsp salt

¼ tsp garlic, minced

1 (grated) big carrot

Freshly ground pepper

10 oz. fresh baby spinach

1 (sliced very thin) medium red bell pepper

Directions

1. Add pepper, salt, garlic, soy sauce, ketchup, ginger, vinegar, oil and onion into a high speed electric blender.

2. Blend mixture until combined.

3. Add bell pepper, carrot and spinach into a big bowl and toss with the blended ginger dressing until wholly coated.

4. Serve and enjoy.

Lime, Olive Anchovy Salad with Orange

Preparation Time: 30 minutes

Cook Time: 0 minutes

Serves: 4 servings

Ingredients

1 (thinly sliced into rounds) small red onion

1/3 tsp ground pepper

3 tbsps olive oil

1 tbsp fresh lime juice

6 anchovy fillets

16 (pitted & halved) salt-cured Kalamata olives

4 small oranges

Garnish with

2 tsps fennel fronds, finely minced

Directions

1. Place oranges on a plate and carefully peel away the white pith and the covering membrane of the oranges, using a paring knife.

2. Slice each peeled orange into very thin rounds as achievable.

3. Place orange rounds on a plate.

TIP: collect orange juice from the plate you used for slice and reserve juice for later use.

4. Lay onion rounds oranges and top with the halved oloves.

5. Add the fish fillets over oranges salad, topped with a generous drizzle of oil, lime juice and orange juice.

6. Sprinkle pepper over salad and let salad sit for about 30 minutes until flavor is infused, at room temperature.

7. Plate salad and sprinkle with fennel fronds to garnish.

Colorful Fruit Salad

Preparation Time: 10 minutes

Cook Time: 0 minutes

Serves: 8 servings

Ingredients

2 cups halved raspberries

2 cups seedless black grapes, halved

2 tbsps purple basil, chopped (if desired)

2 cups plums, diced

Directions

1. If using, add basil with the plums, raspberries and grapes into a big bowl.

2. Stir until combined.

3. Drizzle with desired yogurt salad dressing.

Cole Slaw

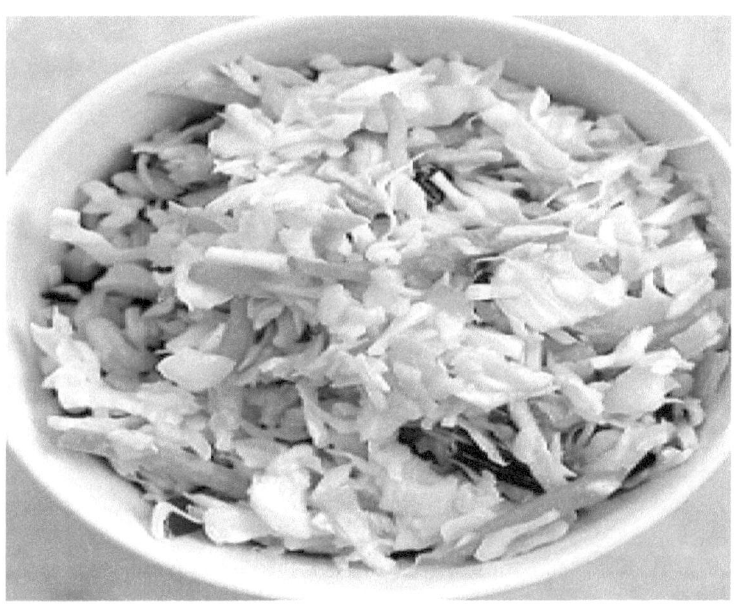

Preparation Time: 15 minutes

Cook Time: 0 minutes

Serves: 6 servings

Ingredients

1 head cabbage, shredded

3 cups shredded raw broccoli

2 tbsps mayonnaise

1/4 cup nonfat Greek yogurt

1 tbsp fresh lime zest

1 tbsp lime juice, freshly squeezed

2 tsps maple syrup

1 tbsp lemon juice

1/8 cup fresh chopped cilantro

1/2 tsp Seasoning Mix (check recipe below)

1 chopped, green onion

Seasoning Mix

1/4 cup garlic powder

1/4 cup pepper

1 cup salt

Directions

1. Add every seasoning mix ingredient into a well lidded bowl and combine.

2. Add shredded cabbage and broccoli into a big bowl.

3. Add 1/2 tsp seasoning mix, maple syrup, lemon juice, lime zest, lime juice, mayonnaise and yogurt into a bowl and whisk until combined.

4. Pour dressing over cabbage mixture and toss until well coated.

5. Add green onions and chopped cilantro and toss until combined.

6. Place plastic wrap over bowl to cover and place in a refrigerator for 60 minutes or more.

7. Serve chilled and enjoy.

Delicious Chickpea Salad

Preparation Time: 10 minutes

Cook Time: 0 minutes

Serves: 4 servings

Ingredients

1 grated carrot

2 (19-oz.) cans {drained & rinsed} chickpeas

1/2 diced green bell pepper

1/2 diced red onion

2 tbsps canola oil

1/4 cup lime juice

Freshly ground black pepper

Salt

1/4 cup mint, freshly chopped

Direction

1. Add every ingredient into a big bowl.

2. Toss until well combined.

3. Serve at once and dig in.

Seafood

Brussels Sprouts with Garlic Roasted Salmon

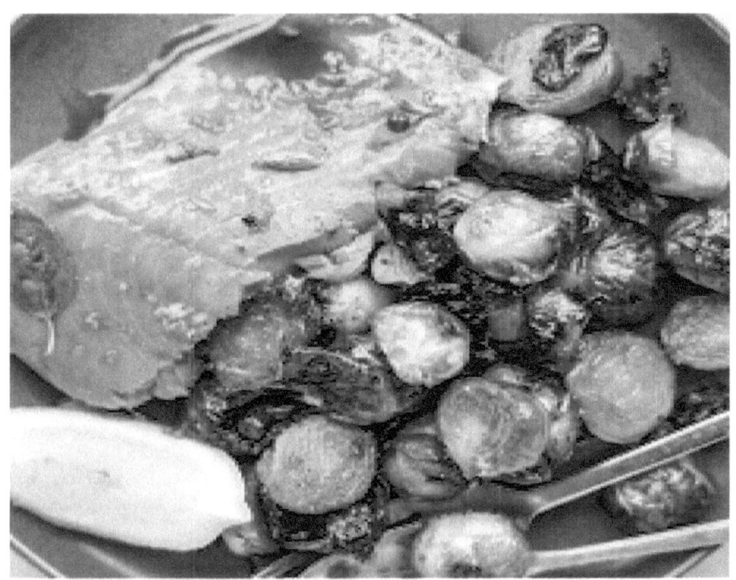

Preparation Time: 10 minutes

Cook Time: 25 minutes

Serves: 6 servings

Ingredients

¼ cup canola oil

12 big garlic cloves (halved)

1 tsp salt (split)

2 tbsps fresh oregano, finely chopped (split)

6 cups (trimmed & sliced) Brussels sprouts

¾ tsp freshly ground pepper (split)

2 lbs. (skinned & cut into 6 portions) wild-caught salmon fillet

¾ cup white wine

2 big garlic cloves, minced

Lime wedges

Directions

1. Heat up oven to 450°F.

2. Add 1/4 tsp pepper, 1/2 tsp salt, 1 tbsp oregano, canola oil and 2 minced garlic cloves into a small bowl and combine.

3. Toss Brussels sprouts with 3 tbsps of the canola oil mixture and the garlic halves until combined.

4. Place seasoned sprouts in a big roasting pan.

5. Place pan into the preheated oven and roast for 15 minutes, stirring once.

6. Add white wine into the remaining canola oil mixture.

7. Take out roasting pan, stir the veggies and add the fish over the sprouts.

8. Drizzle the white wine and canola oil mixture over fish and veggies.

9. Sprinkle with 1/2 tsp pepper, 1/2 tsp salt and the remaining 1 tbsp oregano.

10. Return roasting pan into the oven and bake for 5-10 more minutes, until the fish is cooked through.

11. Serve, garnished with lime wedges.

Bagna Cauda, Veggies with Salmon

Preparation Time: 15 minutes

Cook Time: 25 minutes

Serves: 4 servings

Ingredients

1 bunch (trimmed) broccolini

1 lb. (halved & cut into 1/2" thick wedges) sweet potatoes

½ tsp (split) salt

1 tbsp canola oil

1 (cut into 1/2" thick wedges, reserve fronds) small fennel bulb

1 lb. salmon

½ (sliced into 1/2" thick wedges)

2 medium heads (leaves separated) Belgian endive

Bagna Cauda

2 (sliced very thin) garlic cloves

1/3 cup canola oil

2 tbsps sherry vinegar

8 anchovy fillets

1 tbsp butter

Directions

1. Heat up oven to 425°F.

2. Prepare a big rimmed cooking spray covered baking sheet.

3. Add 1/4 tsp salt, 1 tbsp canola oil, broccolini and sweet potatoes into a big bowl and toss until combined.

4. Let broccolini sit in the bowl, and add the potatoes onto the prepared baking sheet.

5. Place baking sheet into the preheated oven and roast for 15 minutes, flipping halfway while roasting.

6. Push sweet potatoes to the rim of the baking sheet, creating an empty space in the middle.

7. Season salmon with the remaining 1/2 tsp salt and add into the empty space in the middle of the baking sheet.

8. Place pan into the oven and roast for 6-10 minutes, until salmon is cooked through and the veggies are softened.

9. In the meantime, Add oil into a small saucepan over med-low heat.

10. Add garlic into the saucepan and cook for about 2 minutes until aromatic.

11. Add anchovies into the saucepan and crush lightly until they flake apart.

12. Add butter and vinegar into the saucepan and stir cook for 2 more minutes.

13. Plate radicchio, endive, broccolini with fennel, sweet potatoes and salmon and garnish with the reserved fennel fronds.

14. Drizzle with bagna cauda or serve as a dip.

One Pan Garlic Roasted Salmon with Broccoli

Preparation Time: 15 minutes

Cook Time: 15 minutes

Serves: 4 servings

Ingredients

2 heads (washed & cut into about 4 cups of florets) broccoli

1 1/2 lbs. (skinned & cut into 4 portions) salmon fillets

1-2 mince garlic cloves, split

3 tbsps avocado oil

1/2 tsp ground black pepper, split

1 1/4 tsp sea salt, split

1 lime, sliced (if desired)

Directions

1. Heat up oven to 450°F.

2. Prepare a big parchment paper lined baking sheet.

3. Add fish pieces onto the prepared baking sheet and leave out a small amount of space between fish portions.

4. Dribble 1 tbsp avocado oil over salmon pieces and lay the minced garlic cloves over salmon portions until evenly covered.

5. Season salmon with 1/4 tsp black pepper and 1/2 tsp salt.

6. Spread lime slices over fish portions.

7. Add 1/4 tsp ground black pepper, 3/4 tsp sea salt, 2 tbsps oil and washed broccoli florets into a fairly big bowl.

8. Toss the broccoli mixture until wholly coated.

9. Lay seasoned broccoli florets around the fish pieces on the baking sheet.

10. Transfer baking pan into the preheated oven and bake until the edges of the broccoli florets are golden and salmon is cooked through, for 13-15 minutes.

11. Serve warm.

Romaine, Potatoes and Roasted Salmon

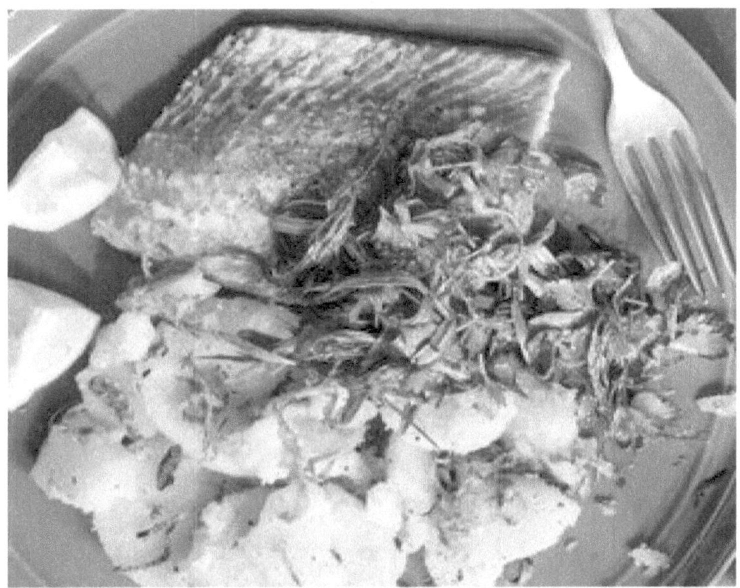

Preparation Time: 10 minutes

Cook Time: 30 minutes

Serves: 4 servings

Ingredients

4 tbsps (split) avocado oil

1 lb. baby potatoes

Salt & freshly ground black pepper to taste

1 tsp lime juice

1 tbsp butter, melted

4 (6-oz.) salmon fillets

2 (slice in half) hearts romaine lettuce

¼ tsp paprika

Directions

1. Heat up oven to 400°F.

2. Add 2 tbsps avocado oil and potatoes into a fairly big bowl and toss until wholly covered.

3. Lay oil coated potatoes on a pre-greased baking sheet.

4. Transfer baking sheet into the preheated oven and roast for 15-20 minutes, until potatoes are fork tender and slightly golden.

5. In the meantime, rub lime juice and 2 tbsps avocado oil over romaine hearts, and liberally season with pepper and salt.

6. Brush melted butter over fish fillet and season with pepper, salt and paprika.

7. Add salmon and romaine into the baking sheet with the partially roasted potatoes.

8. Roast salmon potato mixture until fish is well cooked and romaine is soft, for 5-7 more minutes.

9. Split salmon, romaine and potatoes between 4 plates.

10. Serve and enjoy.

Healthy Rosemary Baked Tilapia

Preparation Time: 15 minutes

Cook Time: 20 minutes

Serves: 4 servings

Ingredients

1/3 cup panko breadcrumbs, whole wheat

1/3 cup raw pecans, chopped

1/2 teaspoon brown sugar

2 teaspoons fresh rosemary, chopped

1 pinch cayenne pepper

1/8 teaspoon salt

1 egg white

1 1/2 teaspoons avocado oil

4 (4 ounce each) tilapia fillets

Directions

1. Heat up oven to 350°F.

2. Add cayenne pepper, salt, brown sugar, rosemary, breadcrumbs and pecans into a small baking dish and stir until combined.

3. Add avocado oil into the crumb mixture and toss until coated.

4. Place crumb mixture in the oven and bake for 7-8 minutes until light golden brown.

5. Adjust oven temperature to 400°F.

6. Prepare a big cooking spray covered glass baking dish.

7. Add egg white into a shallow dish and whisk.

8. Work in batches, immerse tilapia in the egg white and then dip into the rosemary crumb mixture until the fish sides are lightly covered.

9. Transfer coated fish fillets into the prepared baking dish.

10. Add any remaining rosemary crumb mixture over the fillets and press until it sticks.

11. Transfer into the oven and bake for 10 minutes, until fish is well cooked.

12. Serve and enjoy.

Cucumber and Tomato Dressed Salmon

Preparation Time: 10 minutes

Cook Time: 15 minutes

Serves: 4 servings

Ingredients

2 (seed & dice to 1/4" pieces) small plum tomatoes

1/2 (diced into 1/4" pieces) cucumber, seedless

2 tbsps Dijon mustard

1 (finely chopped) shallot, split

1/4 cup white wine vinegar

2 tbsps honey

1/4 cup fresh dill, finely chopped

1/2 cup olive oil

Freshly ground black pepper

Salt

Seafood seasoning

4 (6-oz.) salmon fillets, skinless

Directions

1. Add the tomatoes, cucumber and half of the shallots into a bowl, combine and let sit until needed.

2. Add the remaining half of the shallots, white wine vinegar, honey and mustard into a small bowl and whisk until combined.

3. Slowly add olive oil into the dressing in a steady stream while whisking.

4. Add dill into the dressing and stir until combined.

5. Season dressing with pepper and salt.

6. Season fish fillets with a small amount of black pepper and seafood seasoning.

7. Add olive oil into a nonstick skillet over med-high heat.

8. Add seasoned fish fillets into the skillet with the rounded side facing down and cook for 3-4 minutes until slightly crispy at the edges and golden.

9. Flip fillets and cook until fish is opaque, for 4 minutes.

10. Plate salmon, topped with tomato-cucumber mixture with a generous amount of dressing.

Maple Balsamic Salmon with Brussels Sprouts

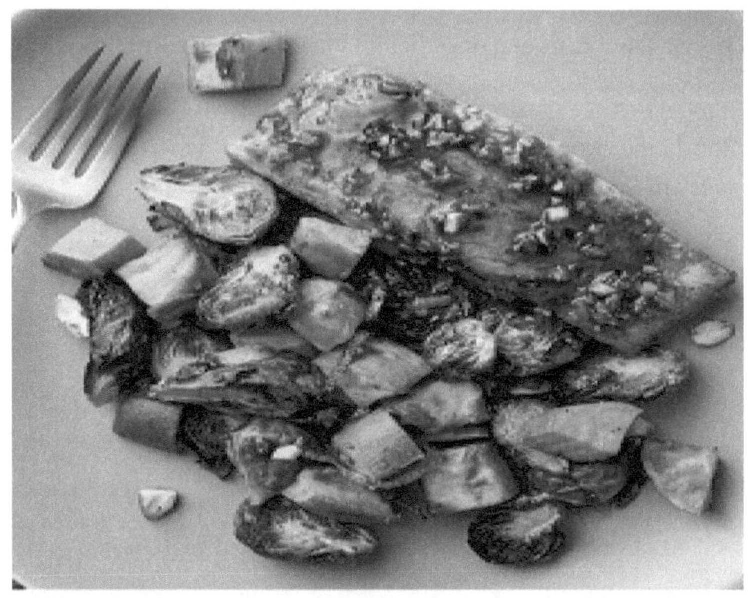

Preparation Time: 5 minutes

Cook Time: 25 minutes

Serves: 4 servings

Ingredients

16 ounces (halved) Brussels sprouts

4 (4-6 ounces) {skin-on} salmon fillets

1 (16 ounce) bag baby potatoes

1 bunch (trimmed & sliced in half) asparagus

1 cup cherry tomatoes

1/2 (cubed) red onion

2 tbsps pure maple syrup

2 tbsps olive oil

1 tbsp dijon mustard

3 tbsps balsamic vinegar

1 tsp fresh thyme

1 minced garlic clove

1/2 tsp sea salt

Directions

1. Heat up oven to 450°F.

2. Add salt, fresh thyme, garlic, dijon mustard, balsamic vinegar and maple syrup into a small bowl and whisk until combined.

3. Add olive oil, cherry tomatoes, red onion, baby potatoes, asparagus and Brussels sprouts into a big bowl.

4. Add 3 tbsps of the maple vinegar mixture into the bowl with the sprouts.

5. Toss veggies with sauce until wholly coated, using clean hands.

6. Spread veggies in on layer on a prepared baking sheet and transfer into the preheated oven.

7. Bake veggies for 10 minutes, take out baking pan and add fish fillets with the skin side down over veggies.

NOTE: Leave room between each fillet- about 1" apart.

8. Brush the maple vinegar sauce over salmon to coat and return baking sheet into the oven.

9. Bake salmon and veggies for 10 more minutes.'

10. Broil salmon for 3-4 minutes on High, until salmon top is browned.

11. Take out of the oven, serve and enjoy.

Broccoli and Quinoa with Orange Salmon

Preparation Time: 10 minutes

Cook Time: 15 minutes

Serves: 4 servings

Ingredients

½ cup orange juice + 1/3 cup, split

1 cup quinoa

8 oz. broccoli florets

2 (sliced) scallions

½ tsp (split) ground pepper

1 tbsp olive oil

¼ tsp garlic powder

3 tsps (split) toasted sesame oil

1 tsp black sesame seeds

4 (4-oz.) portions wild salmon

1 tbsp tamari, reduced-sodium

1 tbsp fresh ginger, minced

1 tsp cornstarch

Directions

1. Add 1/2 cup orange juice and quinoa into a pot over med-heat.

2. Cook quinoa according to instructions on the package.

3. Take quinoa off heat, add the scallions and stir until evenly distributed.

4. Place lid over pot to retain heat.

5. Heat up oven to 450°F.

6. Prepare a rimmed aluminum foil lined baking sheet.

7. Add 1/4 tsp pepper, 1/4 tsp salt and oil over broccoli florets in a big bowl and toss until seasoned.

8. Place seasoned broccoli florets onto the prepared baking sheet.

9. Place baking sheet into the preheated oven and roast for 5 minutes.

10. In the meantime, add the remaining pepper and salt, garlic powder and 2 tsps sesame oil into a small bowl.

11. Brush salmon with the seasoning mix.

12. Push broccoli florets to a side of the baking sheet and add the seasoned salmon to the opposite side.

13. Return baking sheet into the oven and bake for 5-8 minutes until salmon is cooked through.

14. Sprinkle sesame seeds over salmon.

15. Add cornstarch, tamari, ginger, 1 tsp sesame oil and the remaining cup of orange juice into a small oven-secure bowl and whisk until combined.

16. Place bowl in a microwave and heat for a minute, on High.

17. Split salmon, roasted broccoli and quinoa between four serving plates.

18. Drizzle each serving with 2 tbsps orange sauce.

Caramelized Onions and Sardines with Romaine

Preparation Time: 15 minutes

Cook Time: 18 minutes

Serves: 4 servings

Ingredients

1 sliced big sweet onion

1 tbsp canola oil

2 tbsps brown rice vinegar

1/3 tsp salt + ½ tsp

2 tbsps mayo, low-fat

½ cup plain Greek yogurt, low-fat

4 tsps shallot, minced

2 tbsps white wine vinegar

2 (halved lengthways & cored) romaine hearts

¼ tsp freshly ground pepper

1 cup halved grape

2 (4-oz.) cans {drained} bone-in sardines, packed in olive oil

Directions

1. Add oil into a small saucepan over med-heat; add onion and 1/3 tsp salt.

2. Place lid over saucepan and cook for 12-15 minutes until onions are very tender, stirring every now and then.

TIP: If onions are browning too quickly, adjust heat to med-low.

3. Add brown rice vinegar, stir until incorporated and simmer without covering, for about 1-3 minutes, until reduced to a glaze.

4. Add 1/2 tsp salt, pepper, shallow, white wine vinegar, mayo and yogurt into a small bowl and whisk until combined.

5. Split romaine halves between 4 platters, topped with generous scoops of the yogurt dressing.

6. Break each sardine into 2-3 parts.

7. Split sardine between each serving and top with tomatoes and the caramelized onions.

Greens, Chickpeas with Roasted Salmon

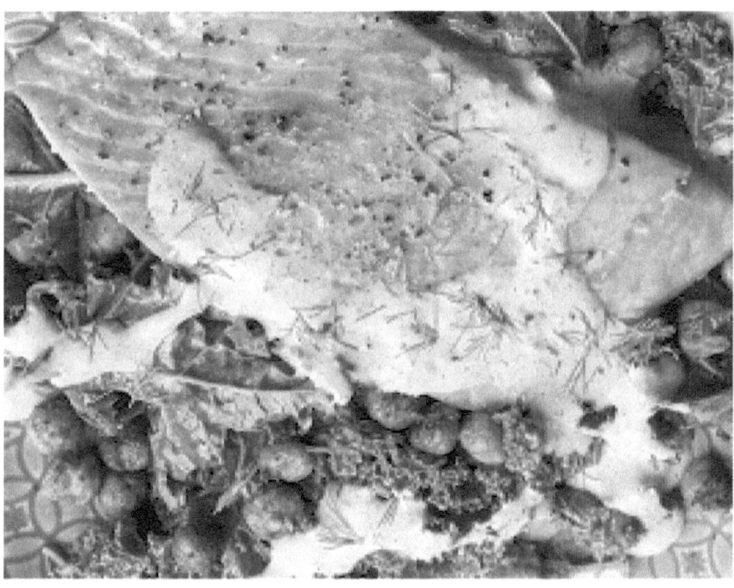

Preparation Time: 10 minutes

Cook Time: 40 minutes

Serves: 4 servings

Ingredients

1 tbsp smoked paprika

2 tbsps (split) olive oil

1 (15 oz.) can {rinsed} chickpeas, no-salt-added

½ tsp (split) salt + a pinch

¼ cup mayo

1/3 cup buttermilk

½ tsp (split) ground pepper

¼ cup fresh chives, chopped

10 cups kale, chopped

¼ tsp garlic powder

1¼ lbs. (cut into 4 portions) wild salmon

¼ cup water

Directions

1. Heat up oven to 425°F.

2. Place racks in the middle and upper third of the oven.

3. Add 1/4 tsp salt, paprika and 1 tbsp oil into a fairly big bowl and combine.

4. Rinse chickpeas and pat dry until well dried.

5. Add chickpeas into the salt mixture and toss until wholly seasoned.

6. Add seasoned chickpeas onto a rimmed baking sheet and spread.

7. Place the baking sheet with chickpeas on the upper third rack and bake for 30 minutes, stirring 2 times.

8. In the meantime, add garlic powder, 1/4 tsp pepper, herbs, mayo and buttermilk into a high speed electric blender.

9. Puree mixture until a smooth consistency is reached.

10. In the meantime, add 1 tbsp oil into a big skillet over med-heat.

11. Add kale into the hot oil and stir cook for 2 minutes.

12. Add water into the skillet and cook for about 5 more minutes until the kale is softened.

13. Take kale off heat, add a pinch of salt and stir until combined.

14. Take out the roasted chickpeas and push to a side of the baking sheet.

15. Season salmon with 1/4 tsp pepper and 1/4 tsp salt until wholly covered.

16. Place seasoned salmon on the empty side of the baking sheet with roasted chickpeas.

17. Return baking sheet into the oven and bake for 5-8 minutes until the fish is cooked through.

18. Serve chickpeas, kale and salmon, drizzled with the blended buttermilk dressing and garnish with herbs, if desired.

Delicious Grilled Mackerel

Preparation Time: 10 minutes

Cook Time: 10 minutes

Serves: 4 servings

Ingredients

1 tbsp olive oil

2 tbsps chile paste

2 tsps rice vinegar

1 tbsp soy sauce, reduced-sodium

2 (1 1/2 lbs. each) {cleaned & butterflied with tails left on} whole mackerel

1 tsp fresh ginger, grated

Directions

1. Add ginger, vinegar, soy sauce, oil and chile paste into a small bowl and whisk until a smooth consistency is reached.

2. Add 2 tbsps of the combined marinade into a separate bowl and keep for later use.

3. Butterfly each fish until the flesh is exposed.

4. Add the butterflied fish onto a baking sheet with the skin side down.

5. Spread the remaining marinade over fish until wholly covered and transfer baking sheet into a refrigerator for 30-60 minutes until marinated.

6. Heat up grill, 20 minutes before cooking.

7. Fold a paper towel and oil, hold the oiled paper towel with tongues and rub over grill rack until well greased.

8. Place fish on the preheated grill with the flesh side down.

9. Grill fish for 3 minutes; turn over using a big spatula and coat with the reserved marinade.

10. Grill fish for 3-4 more minutes until opaque in the middle.

Side

Roasted Garlic Hummus

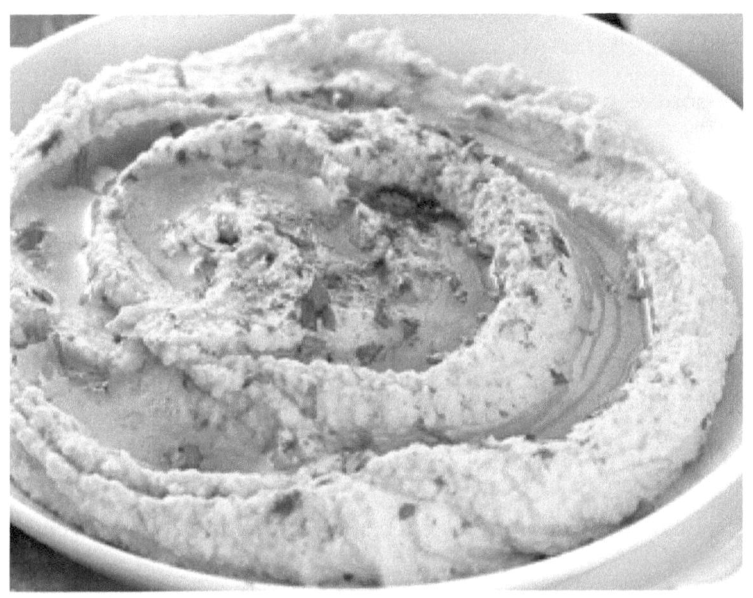

Preparation Time: 10 minutes

Cook Time: 20 minutes

Serves: 6 servings

Ingredients

1 tbsp olive oil + 1 tsp

3 (unpeeled) big garlic cloves

1/4 cup lime juice, freshly squeezed

1 (19-oz.) can {drained} chickpeas

3 tbsps water

3 tbsps sesame tahini

1/4 tsp cayenne pepper

1 tsp coarse salt

1/4 cup fresh minced chives

Serve with

Assorted crudités

Directions

1. Heat up oven to 400°F.

2. Dribble 1 tsp olive oil over garlic cloves.

3. Wrap a small piece of aluminum foil around oiled garlic cloves and seal foil until a pouch is formed.

4. Place in the preheated oven and roast for about 20 minutes until tender.

5. Take out garlic from the oven and let sit until slightly cooled.

6. Peel roasted garlic and place in a food processor.

7. Add chickpeas into the food processor and process with the garlic until a finely chopped consistency is reached.

8. Add 1 tbsp olive oil, cayenne pepper, salt, water, sesame tahini and lime juice into the food processor.

9. Process mixture for about 2 minutes, until a fluffy and light consistency is reached.

TIP: Mixture should not be completely smooth.

10. Add the chives, stir until incorporated and transfer hummus into a serving bowl.

11. Serve with assorted crudités, if you desire.

Chive and Cashew Cream Dip

Preparation Time: 10 minutes

Cook Time: 0 minutes

Serves: 1 cup

Ingredients

1/2 cup water

1 cup (soak overnight) raw cashews

1/2 teaspoon garlic, minced

2 tablespoons fresh lime juice

1/2 teaspoon gray sea salt

1 teaspoon nutritional yeast

1 tablespoon fresh basil, minced

2 tablespoons fresh chives, minced

1 tablespoon fresh dill, minced

Directions

1. Add salt, nutritional yeast, garlic, lime juice, water and cashews into a food processor.

2. Process cashew mixture until a smooth and silky consistency is reached.

TIP: Stop every now and then to scrape food processor insides, using a spatula.

3. Add the dill, basil and chives into the food processor.

4. Process in short pulses to mix in the dill mixture.

5. Place dip in a refrigerator for 30 minutes or more before serving.

Turmeric Tahini Dip with Ginger

Preparation Time: 10 minutes

Cook Time: 0 minutes

Serves: 8 servings

Ingredients

¼ cup rice vinegar

½ cup tahini

1 tbsp fresh ginger, grated

¼ cup water

1 tsp garlic, grated

2 tsps turmeric, ground

½ tsp salt

Directions

1. Add salt, garlic, turmeric, ginger, water, vinegar and tahini into a fairly big bowl.

2. Whisk mixture until combined and a smooth consistency is reached.

3. Serve and enjoy.

Delicious Roasted Beet Hummus

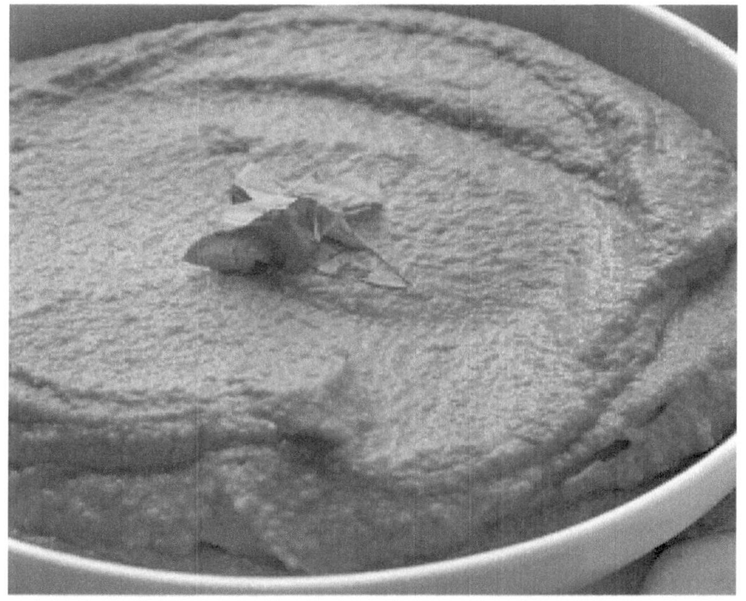

Preparation Time: 10 minutes

Cook Time: 0 minutes

Serves: 10 servings

Ingredients

8 oz. (roughly chopped & pat dried) roasted beets

1 (15 oz.) can {rinsed} chickpeas, no-salt-added

¼ cup canola oil

¼ cup tahini

1 garlic clove

¼ cup lime juice

½ tsp salt

1 tsp ground cumin

Directions

1. Add salt, cumin, garlic, lime juice, oil, tahini, beets and chickpeas into a food processor and combine.

2. Puree chickpea mixture for about 3 minutes, until a smooth consistency is reached.

3. Serve with pita or veggie chips.

Chickpeas with Roasted Cauliflower

Preparation Time: 10 minutes

Cook Time: 25 minutes

Serves: 3-4 servings

Ingredients

1 1/2 cups chickpeas, cooked

1 head (cut into florets) cauliflower

2 minced garlic cloves

3 tbsp olive oil

1 tsp cumin, ground

1 1/2 tsps turmeric, ground

1/2 tsp salt

1 tsp coriander, ground

Garnish with

1/4 cup fresh chopped parsley

Directions

1. Heat up oven to 400°F.

2. Add every ingredient into a big bowl until chickpeas and cauli-florets are wholly coated.

3. Spread cauli-floret mixture onto a big parchment paper lined baking sheet and transfer into the preheated oven.

4. Roast cauli-florets until softened, for about 25 minutes.

5. Serve over quinoa or as a side.

Snacks and Nibble

Cranberry Peanut Trail mix

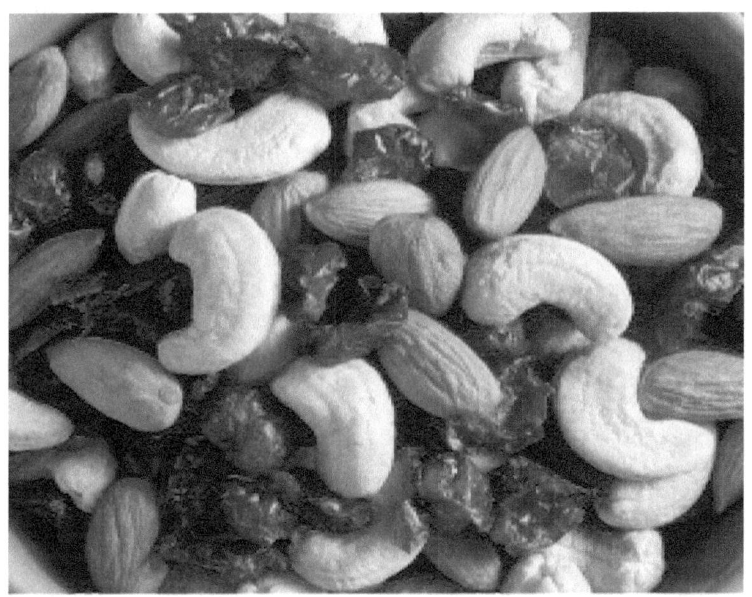

Preparation Time: 5 minutes

Cook Time: 0 minutes

Serves: 5 servings

Ingredients

¼ cup unsalted peanuts, dry-roasted

¼ cup whole shelled almonds, unpeeled

¼ cup dates, pitted & chopped

¼ cup cranberries, dried

2 oz. apricots, dried

Directions

1. Add apricots, dates, cranberries, peanuts and almonds into a fairly big bowl.

2. Mix until combined.

3. Pour into a well lidded container and store at room temperature for up to 14 days.

Healthy Chocolate Trail Mix

Preparation Time: 5 minutes

Cook Time: 0 minutes

Serves: 1 serving

Ingredients

4 apricots, dried

2 tbsps whole almonds

2 tsps dark chocolate chips

Directions

1. Add chocolate chips, apricot and almonds into a bowl.

2. Mix until combined.

3. Serve and enjoy.

Healthy Pistachio Chocolate Kiwi

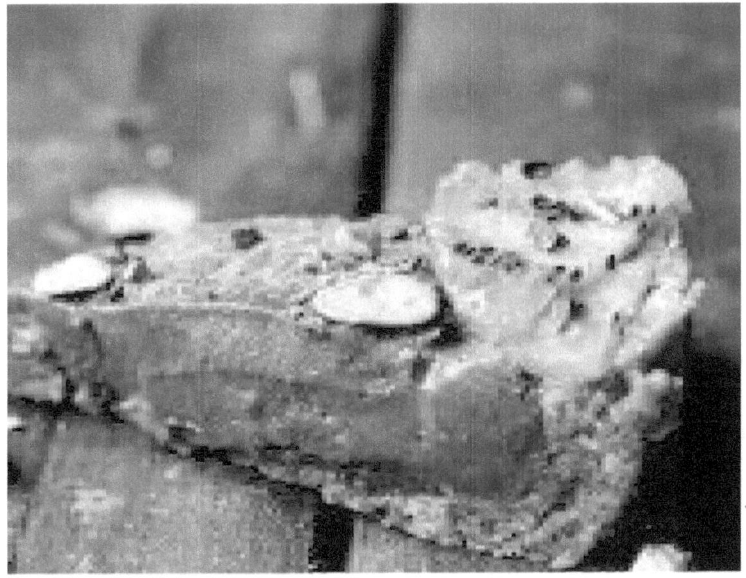

Preparation Time: 5 minutes

Cook Time: 0 minutes

Serves: 1 serving

Ingredients

2 tsps dark chocolate, melted

1 sliced kiwi

1½ tsps salted roasted pistachios, chopped

Directions

1. Add kiwi into a bowl.

2. Drizzle melted dark chocolate over kiwi and top with a generous sprinkle of pistachios.

3. Serve and enjoy.

Cranberry, Raisins and Peanut Snack Mix

Preparation Time: 5 minutes

Cook Time: 0 minutes

Serves: 8 (1/2 cup) servings

Ingredients

1 cup yogurt-covered raisins

1 cup peanuts, lightly salted

1 cup dried cranberries, sweetened

1 cup mini pretzels

Directions

1. Add cranberries, pretzels, raisins and peanuts into a big bowl.

2. Stir mixture until well combined.

3. Store in a well lidded container at room temperature, for up to 2 weeks.

Walnuts and Apricots

Preparation Time: 5 minutes

Cook Time: 0 minutes

Serves: 2 servings

Ingredients

14 walnut halves

10 apricots, dried

Directions

1. Add walnuts and apricot into a container.

2. Toss until combined.

3. Serve and enjoy.

Roasted Chickpeas with Turmeric

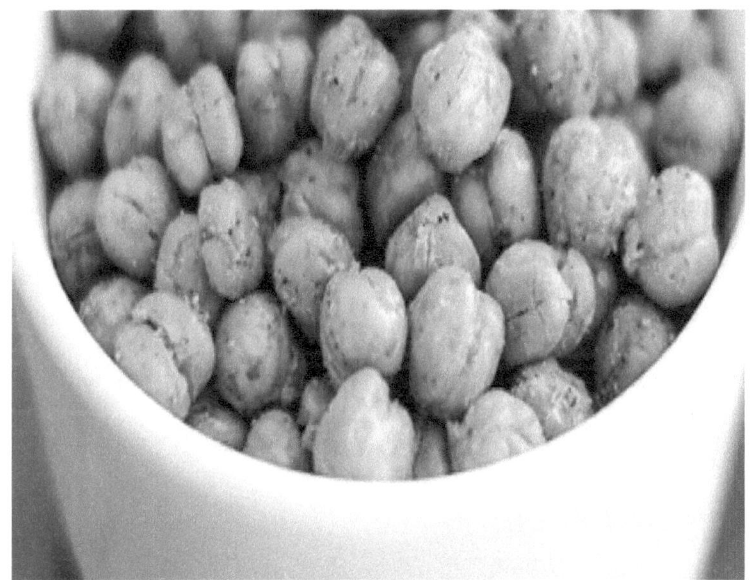

Preparation Time: 10 minutes

Cook Time: 30 minutes

Serves: 15 oz. servings

Ingredients

1/2 tsp paprika

1 tsp turmeric

1 tsp salt

1/4 tsp black pepper

1 can chickpeas, rinsed

2 tsp olive

Directions

1. Heat up oven to 425°F.

2. Prepare a parchment paper lined baking sheet.

3. Add chickpeas and olive oil on the prepared baking sheet and toss until coated.

4. Season chickpeas with spices and salt until wholly covered.

5. Place baking sheet into the preheated oven and bake for 30 minutes.

TIP: Flip pan midway during cooking to ensure that the chickpeas cook evenly.

6. Transfer roasted chickpeas into a well lidded container and store at room temperature.

Soup

Thai Pumpkin Soup

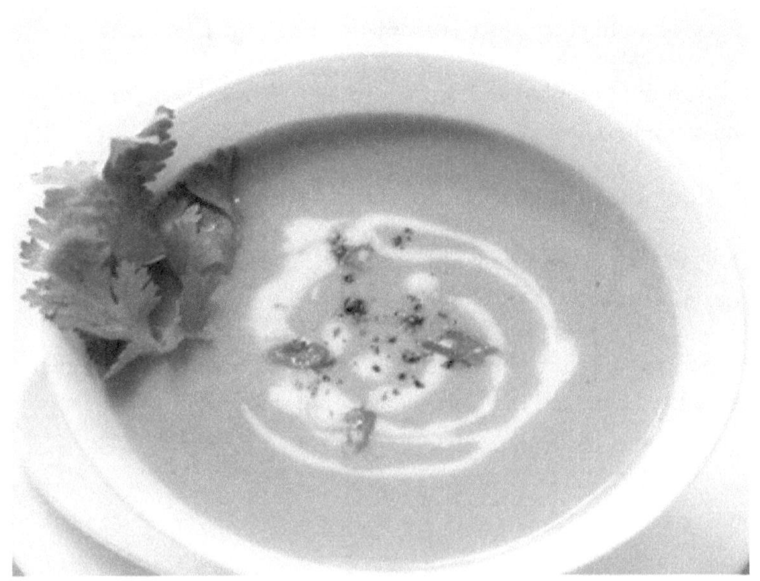

Preparation Time: 10 minutes

Cook Time: 10 minutes

Serves: 4 servings

Ingredients

4 cups veggie broth

2 tbsps red curry paste

1¾ cup coconut milk (keep 1 tbsp coconut milk for garnish)

2 (15 oz.) cans pumpkin puree

1 (sliced) large red chili pepper

Garnish with

Fresh chopped parsley

Directions

1. Add curry paste into a big saucepan over med-heat.

2. Cook until curry paste is aromatic, for about 1 minute.

3. Add the pumpkin and broth into the saucepan and stir until incorporated.

4. Cook soup until bubbly, for about 3 minutes.

5. Add the coconut milk into the soup and cook for about 3 minutes until heated through.

6. Scoop soup into serving bowls, garnished with fresh chopped parsley, sliced red chili and the reserved coconut milk.

7. Serve and enjoy.

Slow Cooked Chicken Chili

Preparation Time: 10 minutes

Cook Time: 4-6 hours

Serves: 8-10 servings

Ingredients

1-pound ground chicken, 99% lean

1 tbsp avocado oil

1 chopped red pepper

1 diced medium onion

2 (15 ounces) cans tomato sauce

1 chopped yellow pepper

2 (15 ounces) cans {rinsed & drained} black beans

2 (15 ounces) cans petite diced tomatoes

1 (16 ounces) jar {drained} deli-sliced tamed jalapeno peppers

2 (15 ounces) cans {rinsed & drained} red kidney beans

2 tbsps chili powder

1 cup corn, frozen

Salt and black pepper

1 tbsp cumin

Top with {if desired}

Greek yogurt

Avocado

Shredded cheese

Green onions

Directions

1. Add avocado oil into a skillet over med-heat.

2. Add ground chicken into the hot oil and saute until chicken is browned.

3. Add ground chicken into a slow cooker pot.

4. Add cumin, chili powder, corn, jalapenos, beans, diced tomatoes, tomato sauce, peppers, and onions into the slow cooker pot.

5. Season with pepper and salt.

6. Stir to combine, place lid over slow cooker and cook for 6 hours on low, or 4 hours on high.

7. Serve with desired toppings.

Turmeric Bok Choy Soup with Shrimp

Preparation Time: 20 minutes

Cook Time: 30 minutes

Serves: 4 servings

Ingredients

1 chopped large onion

1 tbsp olive oil

1 1/2 tsp salt

6 minced garlic cloves

1 tsp turmeric

1 tsp ground black pepper

2 sliced carrots

6 cups chicken broth

6 heads (chop bottoms off) baby bok choy

1 lb. (remove stems, & slice into 1/2" pieces) shitake mushrooms

1 lb. shrimp

Directions

1. Add olive oil into a stock pot over med-heat.

2. Add garlic and onions into the pot and saute until translucent, for 5 minutes.

3. Add mushrooms, carrots, chicken broth, turmeric, pepper and salt into the pot and bring to boiling.

4. Lower heat, place lid over pot and simmer for soup for 15 minutes.

5. Add shrimp and bok choy into the soup and simmer for 5 more minutes.

6. Season soup with pepper and salt, serve and enjoy.

Avocado & White Chicken Chili

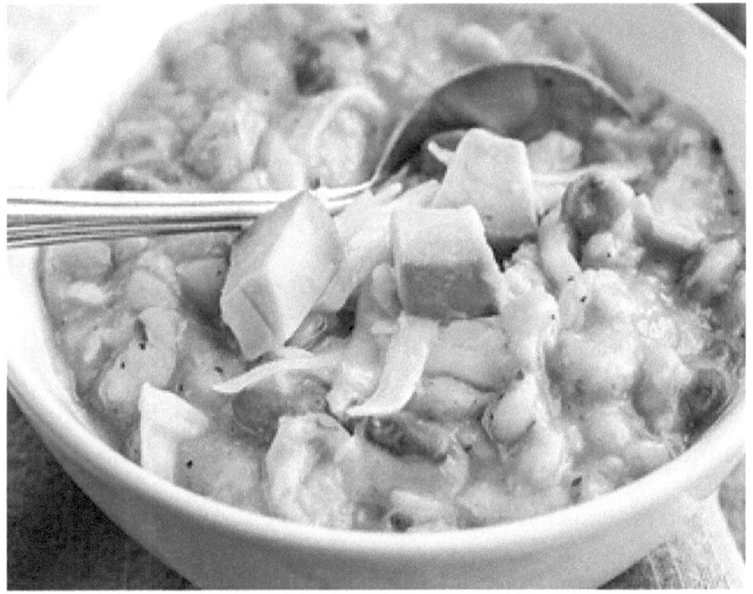

Preparation Time: 5 minutes

Cook Time: 55 minutes

Serves: 8 servings

Ingredients

1 diced large white onion

2 tbsps olive oil

1 lb. ground chicken

4 minced garlic cloves

1 tsp coriander, ground

2 tsps cumin, ground

Salt & freshly ground black pepper

1 tsp cayenne pepper

1 (15-oz.) can corn kernels

4 cups chicken broth

1 diced avocado

1 (15-oz.) can white beans

Directions

1. Add olive oil into a big pot over med-heat.

2. Add onions into the hot oil and saute for 6-8 minutes, until translucent.

3. Add garlic into the onion and oil mixture and cook for a minute until aromatic.

4. Add ground chicken into the oil mixture and cook for 5-7 minutes until well cooked and browned.

5. Add pepper, salt, cayenne, coriander and cumin into the pot and cook for 1-2 minutes until aromatic.

6. Add the broth into the pot and stir until incorporated.

7. Bring soup to simmering over med-heat, adjust heat to low heat and simmer for 30-35 minutes, until flavors are infused.

8. Add beans and corn into chili, stir until incorporated and simmer for 2-3 minutes.

9. Scoop chili into serving bowls, topped 1-2 tbsps avocado dices.

10. Serve at once and dig in.

Squash Red Lentil Curry Stew

Preparation Time: 5 minutes

Cook Time: 25 minutes

Serves: 4 servings

Ingredients

1 chopped sweet onion

1 teaspoon olive oil

1 tablespoon curry powder

3 minced garlic cloves

1 cup red lentils

4 cups low-sodium chicken broth

1 cup greens of choice

3 cups butternut squash, cooked

1/2 teaspoon kosher salt

Fresh ginger, grated

Freshly ground black pepper, to taste

Directions

1. Add olive oil into a big pot over med-low heat.

2. Add minced garlic and chopped onion into the pot and sauté for 5 minutes.

3. Add curry powder into the mixture, stir until combined and cook for few minutes.

4. Add lentils and broth into the pot, adjust heat to med-heat and bring to boiling.

5. Lower heat and cook for about 10 minutes

6. Add in greens of choice and cooked butternut squash, and stir until evenly distributed.

7. Adjust heat to med-heat, and cook for about 5-8 minutes.

8. Add in freshly grated ginger and season lentil mixture with pepper and salt.

9. Serve and enjoy.

White Bean and Turkey Chili Blanca

Preparation Time: 20 minutes

Cook Time: 60 minutes

Serves: 8-10 servings

Ingredients

2 tbsps avocado oil

1 lb. (boneless & skinless) turkey breasts

2 garlic cloves

1 diced medium onion

1 cup fresh corn kernels

2 (15-oz.) cans {drained & rinsed} white beans

2 tsps cumin, ground

1 (4-oz.) can green chiles, chopped

1/8 tsp cayenne pepper

2 tsps pure chili powder

2 cups Monterey Jack cheese, grated

3 cups water

2 tbsps fresh chopped parsley

Directions

1. Sprinkle pepper and salt over turkey until well seasoned.

2. Add avocado oil into a big saucepan over high heat.

3. Add the seasoned turkey pieces into the oil and stir cook for 2-3 minutes until browned.

4. Adjust heat to med-heat, add garlic and onion into saucepan and cook for 5-6 minutes until onion is translucent.

5. Add water, spices, chilies, corn and beans into the saucepan, bring to boiling.

6. Adjust heat to low-heat and simmer chili without covering for 60 minutes.

7. Serve into bowls, and top each bowl with a generous sprinkle of parsley and a spoonful of cheese.

Lentil Veggie Soup

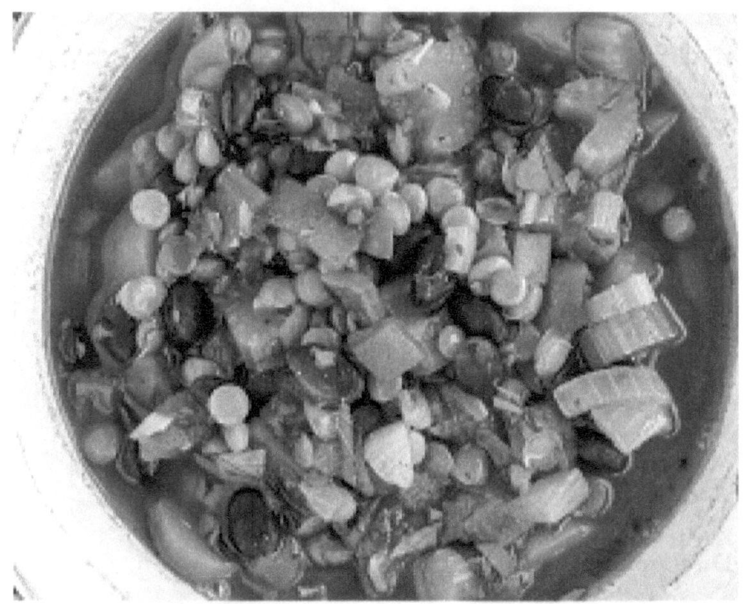

Preparation Time: 20 minutes

Cook Time: 1 hour 30 minutes

Serves: 8-10 servings

Ingredients

4 cups yellow onions, chopped

1 lb. French dry green lentils

1 tbsp garlic cloves, minced

4 cups leeks, white part only {chopped}

1 tbsp kosher salt

1/4 cup avocado oil

1 tbsp fresh thyme leaves, minced

1-½ tsps black pepper, freshly ground

3 cups celery (medium-diced)

1 tsp cumin, ground

3 qts. chicken stock

3 cups carrots (medium-diced)

2 tbsps red wine vinegar

1/4 cup tomato paste

Parmesan cheese, freshly grated

Directions

1. Add lentils and just enough boiling water to cover into a big bowl and set aside until soaked for 15 minutes.

2. Drain off water.

3. Add cumin, thyme, pepper, salt and avocado oil into a big stockpot over med-heat.

4. Add garlic, leeks and onions into the pot and saute until the veggies are softened and translucent, for 20 minutes.

5. Add carrots and celery into the pot and saute for 10 more minutes.

6. Add lentils, tomato paste and chicken stock into the pot, place lid over pot and bring mixture to boiling.

7. Adjust heat to low-heat, remove lid and simmer until the lentils are well cooked, for 1 hour.

8. Check for seasoning, and adjust as necessary.

9. Stir in red wine vinegar, sprinkle with grated Parmesan and drizzle with avocado oil.

10. Serve and enjoy.

Turmeric Carrot Therapeutic Soup with Ginger

Preparation Time: 5 minutes

Cook Time: 15 minutes

Serves: 2 servings

Ingredients

1 (peeled & chopped) parsnip

4 (peeled & chopped) carrots

4 crushed garlic cloves

1 (coarsely chopped) yellow onion

3 cups warm veggie broth, low sodium

2 tsps olive oil

1" (peeled & grated) ginger knob

1 tsp turmeric powder

1 pinch cayenne pepper

1/2 lime, juiced

Serve with

Coconut flakes

Black sesame

Greek yogurt

Fresh chopped cilantro

Directions

1. Heat up oven to 350°F.

2. Prepare a parchment paper lined baking sheet.

3. Add garlic, onion, parsnip and carrots into the prepared baking sheet and season with cayenne and turmeric.

4. Dribble olive oil over carrots mixture and toss until wholly coated.

5. Place in the preheated oven and roast for 15 minutes.

6. Take out baking pan from the oven; pour carrot mixture into a high speed electric blender.

7. Add ginger, lime juice and veggie broth into the blender.

8. Blend carrot soup until a creamy and smooth consistency is reached.

9. Add blended carrot soup into bowls and garnish with coconut flakes, sesame, fresh cilantro and a generous drizzle of Greek yogurt.

Spicy Lentil Soup

Preparation Time: 15 minutes

Cook Time: 20 minutes

Serves: 7 cups

Ingredients

2 cups onion, diced

1 1/2 tbsps olive oil

2 tsps turmeric, ground

2 minced large garlic cloves

1/2 tsp cinnamon

1 1/2 tsps cumin, ground

1 (15-oz.) can {with juices} diced tomatoes

1/4 tsp cardamom, ground

3/4 cup {rinsed & drained} uncooked red lentils

1 (15-oz.) can coconut milk, full-fat

1/2 tsp fine sea salt, as needed

3 1/2 cups veggie broth, low-sodium

Cayenne pepper, as needed

Freshly ground black pepper, as needed

2 tsps fresh lemon juice

1 (5-oz.) package baby spinach

Directions

1. Add garlic, onion and oil into a big pot over med-heat.

2. Season with a pinch of salt and stir until incorporated.

3. Saute onion mixture until onion is tenderized, for 4-5 minutes.

4. Add cardamom, cinnamon, cumin and turmeric into the pot and stir until incorporated.

5. Keep cooking until aromatic for about 1 more minute.

6. Add a liberal amount of pepper, salt, broth, red lentils, coconut milk and the diced tomatoes with juices.

7. Add cayenne pepper into the soup and stir until well combined.

8. Adjust heat to high heat and bring mixture to low boiling.

9. Readjust heat to med-high heat; simmer without covering until lentils are softened and fluffy, for about 18-22 minutes.

10. Turn off the heat, add the spinach, stir until well combined and let sit until spinach wilts.

11. Add lemon juice into soup and check for seasoning and adjust pepper and salt, if necessary.

12. Stir to combine and scoop soup in bowl.

13. Eat alone or serve with toasted bread and lemon wedges.

Turmeric Garlic Carrot Soup

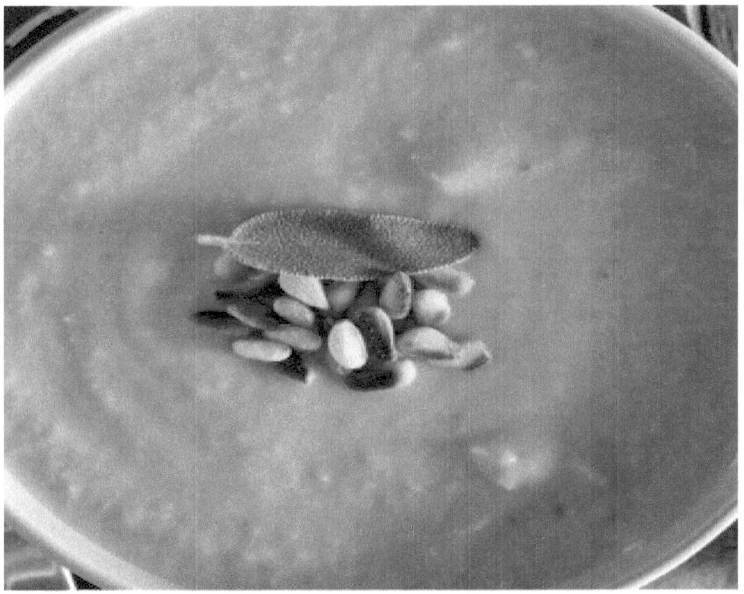

Preparation Time: 15 minutes

Cook Time: 30 minutes

Serves: 4 servings

Ingredients

1 (diced into small chunks) white onion

3 (diced into small chunks) carrots

1" piece (finely grated) fresh ginger

3 minced garlic cloves

4 cups veggie stock

2" piece (finely grated) fresh turmeric

1 tablespoons lime juice

Top with

Black sesame seeds

Coconut milk

Directions

1. Add avocado oil into a big stock pot over med-heat.

2. Add onion into the hot oil and saute until translucent for 3 minutes.

3. Add ginger, turmeric and minced garlic into the pot and saute for a minute.

4. Add the diced carrot into the ginger mixture and saute for 2 more minutes.

5. Add the veggie stock into the pot and simmer until the carrot is tender and well cooked, for 20-25 minutes.

6. Blend carrot soup until a smooth and creamy consistency is reached, using an immersion blender.

7. Add lime juice into the soup and stir until evenly distributed.

8. Serve, topped with black sesame seeds and a liberal swirl coconut milk.

Sweet Potato with Roasted Red Pepper Soup

Preparation Time: 25 minutes

Cook Time: 30 minutes

Serves: 6 servings

Ingredients

2 chopped, medium onions

2 tbsps avocado oil

1 (4 ounces) can green chiles, diced

1 (12 ounces) jar (chopped, reserve liquid) roasted red peppers

1 tsp salt

2 tsps cumin, ground

3–4 cups sweet potatoes, peeled & cubed

1 tsp coriander, ground

2 tbsps minced fresh parsley

4 cups veggie broth

4 ounces (cubed) cream cheese

1 tbsp lime juice

Directions

1. Add avocado oil into a big soup pot over med-high heat.

2. Add onions into the hot oil and cook until the onions are tenderized.

3. Add coriander, salt, cumin, green chiles and red pepper into the pot and cook for 1-2 more minutes.

4. Add the veggie broth, sweet potatoes and the reserved roasted red pepper juice into the pot and stir until combined.

5. Bring mixture to boiling, lower heat and place lid over pot.

6. Cook potatoes for 10-15 minutes until softened.

7. Add lime juice and fresh chopped parsley and stir until incorporated.

8. Let soup sit until slightly cooled before using an immersion blender to puree until desired consistency is reached.

9. Check for seasoning and adjust salt as necessary.

Ginger Carrot Soup

Preparation Time: 10 minutes

Cook Time: 10 minutes

Serves: 6 cup servings

Ingredients

4 tsps ginger, minced

1/4 cup shallots, minced

1 lb. (peeled & chopped) carrots

2 tbsps coconut oil

4 cups water

1 (peeled & chopped) medium sweet potato

Yogurt

Coarse salt

Directions

1. Add coconut oil into a pot over med-heat.

2. Add ginger and shallots into the oil and cook for 2 minutes, until aromatic.

3. Add 2 tsps sea salt, water, sweet potato and carrots into the pot, place lid over pot and simmer for 10 minutes until the veggies are softened.

4. Pour mixture into a high speed electric blender.

5. Blend mixture until a smooth consistency is reached.

6. Serve immediately or let sit until cooled before serving, top with yogurt.

END

Thank you for reading my book.

Stephanie Trask

www.ingramcontent.com/pod-product-compliance
Lightning Source LLC
Chambersburg PA
CBHW021138260726
48656CB00023B/323